HOW TO MAKE
GREAT LOVE
TO A MAN

Also by Phillip Hodson and Anne Hooper

How to Make Great Love to a Woman

HOW TO MAKE GREAT LOVE TO A MAN

PHILLIP HODSON AND ANNE HOOPER

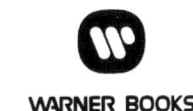

WARNER BOOKS

An AOL Time Warner Company

To Terry Mansfield,
with love

Warner Books Edition

This Warner Books edition is published by arrangement with
Robson Books, 10 Blenheim Court, Brewery Road, London N7 9NT

Visit our Web site at www.twbookmark.com.

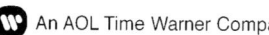 An AOL Time Warner Company

Printed in Canada
Originally published in hardcover by Robson Books
First Warner Books Printing: June 2002
10 9 8 7 6 5 4 3 2 1

Library of Congress Cataloging-in-Publication Data
Hodson, Phillip.
    How to make great love to a man / Phillip Hodson and Anne Hooper.—Warner Books ed.
        p. cm.
    Originally published: London : Robson Books, 2000.
    Includes bibliographical references.
    ISBN 0-446-67835-X
    1. Sex instruction for women. 2. Women—Sexual behavior. 3. Men—Physiology. 4.
Communication in sex. I. Hooper, Anne, 1941 - II. Title.

HQ46 .H63 2002
613.9'6—dc21

                                                                            2001046555

Photography by John Freeman
Art Direction and Styling by Jack Buchan
Illustrations by Stuart Miller

contents

Preface

'Sex is different for women. They only have to turn up'
– Jackie Mason.

This book is a lover's guide to the male sex for women who want to enjoy and understand their partners. At the start of a new millennium, the direction of male sexuality remains a puzzle. How do we explain some of the contradictions? To pick a few straws from winds in recent years, we have:

- Filmstar Hugh Grant arrested in a car in the arms of a stranger when he apparently had one of the world's most attractive partners available at home. Most women cannot understand his motive in choosing risky novelty over domestic intimacy.
- President Bill Clinton shamed and nearly impeached for seeking superficial orgasms in a corridor with a co-worker. Many are puzzled that fellatio could be worth jeopardising the world's most powerful job.
- Grandfatherly rock singer Mick Jagger beating a Casanova rhythm in the bedrooms of several actresses and models young enough to be his daughters. Some observers wonder whether he may be suffering from a psychological illness such as sex addiction. Others say it's glandular!

NOVELTY AND REASSURANCE

Or, consider some of men's confusions about their gender. In every major Western country – England, France, Germany, Italy and the USA – there is now a small army of transsexual and transvestite prostitutes servicing what seem to be heterosexual men. Does this signpost anything about men's innate sexual desires and fears? Could it be that what men actually want from women is the paradox of a 'man's mind in a woman's body'? Does this mean that men want the prize of novelty wrapped in the ribbon of emotional safety?

If this **is** the case, then this is something else women need to understand. But a word of comfort at the outset – use this book wisely and well and a complete meeting of minds and bodies can still be achieved, whatever men's erratic behaviour. Before we look at ways to greater sexual pleasure, take these facts to heart as well:

- ❦ Two thirds of all marriages last for life.
- ❦ As men and women grow older, they grow more similar. This is even true physically – male faces soften and women's become sturdier with the years.
- ❦ Men's sexual drive is not that of a dinosaur – it is controlled by the forebrain – they can choose to be true and loyal when they want.
- ❦ Men fall in love more easily and out of love with more difficulty than women.
- ❦ When women do get the sex 'right' with their partners, relationships nearly always flourish so you can control your joint destinies.

However, as a broad generalisation, men probably do operate more often in 'emotional compartments' than women. Although they have the same feelings, they find it difficult to label them. The obvious result is that women need to realise how significantly the male sexual imagination **is** different from theirs in order to manage it. To list examples:

- ❦ More men would take sex from a stranger than the average woman would.
- ❦ More men use pornography.

- More men are anxious about sexual performance and prowess than most women are.
- Men use risk both to increase their sexual drive and reinforce it.
- Men are on average both kinkier and apparently less faithful.

Men also realise that their largest sexual organ is the brain. The trouble is that they would secretly like to find their brains in their shorts. Through the centuries, men have been conditioned to lust after women who look young and beautiful. So if you want your love and lust to endure you must probe beneath the surface of these male preferences. Men need reminding by subtle currents of female influence that looks are additional to sexuality and sexuality depends on what happens after you talk. Real lovemaking comes from feelings of attachment to another person as much as the excitement of touching youthful skin. The poet Milton called beauty 'Nature's brag' because it always fades. You need to help your man discover the basic psychic similarities and compatibilities you share together before his time runs out.

However, men are not creatures from Mars. There is no future in treating them with silent contempt. But you do need to accept that the male is writing a slightly different erotic shopping list. Men go from sex into love more often than love into sex. Men trust more slowly and disclose their emotions at higher cost. Men are sexually split – they know sex can be used to make love but believe it represents a pretty good end in itself. As one of the women characters in a Woody Allen film says: 'Sex without love is an empty experience'. 'Yes,' replies Allen, 'but as empty experiences go it's one of the best.' This is how men are in practically all societies. You need to work with and around it till the problem subsides. Sometimes men just want to come – it's safe, really quite harmless. The family pets will not be frightened. You need to realise that sex can be so simple.

And when you do, you must adjust some of your own idealised fantasies. Accepting a man for himself means you probably can't project the childlike dreams of lifetime romantic rescue onto one chap. You may tell yourself, like Mrs Blissfully Innocent: 'He totally loves, supports and adores me'. But he is also bound to fancy looking at other naked women. And at some point in your future he will possibly consider going to bed with one of them. You'd be better prepared if you built this knowledge into your personal understanding. Because that's how men are.

And yet the key to preserving any monogamous harmony also lies in a greater emphasis on exploring your mutual erotic ties. If a man is lucky enough to live with a woman who re-invents her love skills to suit his different ages and stages – who is the proverbial harlot in the bedroom but good companion in the living room – he has no practical incentive to explore his deceitful capacities. Nature will out, but our message is that men can be tamed. And this is the manual.

Phillip Hodson

1

f MEN ARE NOT from MARS

There is no limit to the pleasure you can enjoy except the power of your own imagination. But if this book contains the best of all possible sensual and sexual experiences a woman can give a man, a sensory ideal, how do you set about understanding and creating the circumstances which will make it happen in *your* house for You and Yours? How do you get from ideal to real? We start with the basic male psychology of Chapter One – it's *no* help to imagine that men are from Mars!

PEOPLE ARE ... FROM EARTH

No one today thinks men and women are emotionally identical. John Gray's best-seller *Men are from Mars Women are from Venus* has made this crystal clear. But the two sexes remain different, not oppo-site. If you believe the exaggerations of writers like John Gray you are likely to make good sex much harder to achieve. You will certainly never successfully reconcile your differences. Men and women are *not* alien species from separate worlds. They are similar creatures endeavouring to solve their problems from slightly different viewpoints. This is where we believe John Gray gets it wrong about psychology:

- The differences *within* one sex are far greater than the differences *between* the two sexes. By this we mean that man has wide variations of desire, romance and sexual performance just like woman but that the majority of men and women respond similarly. So it's not true that your lover is on another planet on a different wavelength and unable to 'speak your language'. There will always be major areas where the two of you easily connect if you recognise this and know how to achieve the connection.

- Most psychological surveys show there are *no* major differences between the sexes. But these surveys don't get published because they have 'nothing to report'. The similarities are many. The physiological pattern of sexual response is identical and the hormonal system, despite differing ratios of the sex hormones, works similarly. The sex problems, when they crop up, are physiologically alike. Men suffer from impotence. So, too, do women.

In other words 'People are from Earth'.

Having made this point, it may appear odd to explore the differences that remain. But knowing where men and women are likely to see things as separate systems comes in useful when gauging your own behaviour with your man. The sex differences *that count* are the subject of this chapter. We begin by looking at the ways in which a man's sexual emotions are not quite like yours.

THE PSYCHO-SEXUAL DIFFERENCES

Men's minds work a shade differently from women's, with less acute emotional radar. As a result, they sometimes tend to imagine that girls are like boys with breasts. Where women can be generous to men's physical imperfections and are mainly turned off by their emotional failings, men tend to undervalue the human context in which sex is supplied.

'I don't mind if a woman fails to appreciate me emotionally,' says the Martin Clunes character in the soap *opera Men Behaving Badly*, 'so long as she still gets her kit off.'

Men even regard sex like food. Their characteristic reaction to refusal of sex is puzzlement: 'Why is she on a hunger strike? We all need to eat to survive.' Hence men's propensity to divorce their 'needs' from feelings. As the husband in one Roddy Doyle novel says to his wife immediately after a row: 'I suppose a ride is out of the question?' In seeking comfort, men still solicit sex.

Men pretend to be ever-ready like the battery but are just as likely to have the headaches. They also like to reinforce their own masculine stereotypes. However, contrary to myth, the world is full of hot accountants and cold pop-stars. Despite what men like to think, the sexes are identical in their distribution of desire. A few people have extreme sexual appetites (great or small) while the rest of us come somewhere in the middle.

In terms of sheer appetite, women are apt to be discreet about their amours. Men make propaganda out of theirs. In fact the only way to make any sense of the research on infidelity is to assume that women routinely lie about their lovers. Either that, or one urban sex worker in the North of England is having more partners than hot dinners.

Present psychological thinking, based on many areas of enquiry, accepts the possibility that there is indeed a 'male brain'. This male brain is generally accepted by the female of the species to be:

- less socially clever
- less able to manoeuvre and negotiate within social and emotional relationships
- less able to make the deep and meaningful interpersonal connections that women find so necessary to their own sense of self-worth and well-being.

Whether or not this current research proves fruitful remains to be seen. And even if this current research does not, it's worth remembering that publishing itself is a form of social conditioning. Both sexes are persuaded by books like *Men are from Mars Women are from Venus* to believe that men don't comprehend emotions.

'Men avoid emotional
conflicts by …
withdrawing. As long as the
withdrawal doesn't lead to
long periods of loneliness,
they usually feel just fine
about it. Whether he …
plays computer games,
jogs or just drives around,
the man's main purpose is
to escape the emotional
roller-coaster. It's a self-
protective act. If you ask a
male stonewaller to
describe his state of mind
he often says "I'm trying
not to react". He feels like
he's idling in neutral even
though his wife perceives
his silence as hostility.'

MEN GET FLOODED

The male brain has one further crucial difference from a woman's. Because men tend not to probe into their own or other people's feelings, they are more emotionally vulnerable. According to psychologist Dr John Gottman, men have a stronger physical reaction to all their emotions than women do. If either sex wants to claim the world title for emotions, men could probably do so. In general, there's overwhelming evidence to show men have shorter fuses and suffer longer-lasting explosions when angry.

For example, during a difficult marital row a man's heart rate and blood pressure will rise sharply and stay at an elevated level far longer than his wife's. Typically, the male heart rate will surge to an extra 20 to 30 beats per minute. Sometimes the rate will approach that of a man driving a Formula 1 racing car. This happens swiftly so that he's still stuck with an accelerated heart rate long after the woman has moved on to other subjects. The average woman's rate, by contrast, can stay relatively unchanged before, during and after the 'discussion'. She is apparently more comfortable verbalising her difficulties than avoiding them.

Such gender differences, says Gottman in his book *Why Marriages Succeed or Fail*, help to clarify why men are so much more likely than women to become stonewallers – indeed may even deny that they have emotional difficulties. Gottman suggests that 85 per cent of stonewallers are male and that the purpose of their emotional denials is to protect the male brain from unacceptably high levels of stress.

SAME PROBLEM, DIFFERENT SOLUTIONS

- Men and women identify different points of friction when a relationship begins to fail. Men talk about things like money and sex, women about commitment and intimacy issues.

- Men are far more likely to see the difficulty as a technical hitch rather than a crisis.

- When men stonewall, women generally escalate their demands for a more emotional response.

- As a last resort, women tend to 'throw in the kitchen-sink' – dragging up every single past occasion on which a partner has failed to satisfy them.

- Men interpret this as a declaration of war – often voting with their feet.

HOW TO ARGUE WITHOUT RUINING YOUR RELATIONSHIP

- The magic 5 to 1 ratio: make sure there is five times as much positive feeling between you and your partner as there is negative

- Remove blame from your comments

- Say how you feel

- Listen to your partner

- Don't criticise or try to analyse your partner's personality

- Don't insult, mock or use sarcasm

- Be direct and stick to one situation, rather than dragging up the past

- Learn how to calm yourself when floods of emotion block communication

- Discuss how you can take a break

- Try to think of your partner's good qualities – praise and admire them

- Look at these principles again and again. It takes a long time to learn new habits

DR JOHN GOTTMAN AGAIN

'In happy relationships there are no gender differences in emotional expression. But in unhappy relationships all the gender differences emerge – men are more defensive; men try to keep the emotion on a neutral track but women don't; men are the big stonewallers, withdrawing from the negative emotions of their wives because they are more easily flooded. And the men's withdrawal and defensiveness just fan the flames of their partners' frustration.'

The mathematics of domestic rows simply ensures that more stress is created for the woman because the problems remain unsolved. His gain (when he doesn't have to face up to things) is her loss (since she cannot make him engage with her concerns). Gottman has identified stonewalling as 'the single most destructive behaviour to be found in any modern marriage'. Following a domestic row, and because they are by nature more aggressive, men tend to play negative scripts over and over thus keeping themselves on the boil for far longer and they end up saying to themselves: 'I shouldn't have to take this crap – it's all your fault!'

ARE NORMAL MEN ALMOST BRAIN-DAMAGED?

One real and critical sex difference affecting all our romantic encounters is women's sharper ability to 'read minds'. When a woman looks into your eyes she is better able to tell what you're feeling than the average man. She is more intuitive, quicker to interpret body language, tone of voice even facial expression. The extreme state of psychological withdrawal called autism, associated with a total inability to work out what somebody else is feeling, is much more common in men than in women.

As we know, most babies start life as emotional 'tyrants'. They don't care what other people need – they want attention and will make a fuss if they don't get it. By the age of two, however, toddlers can generally appreciate that different people have different wants and desires but they still cannot understand why.

By the age of five or six, children can tell that different people interpret the world differently and by this stage all children should have become psychologists. The problem is that many boys do not make this leap and a significant proportion of males remains unable to 'think themselves into the shoes of another person'.

Research, led by Simon Baron-Cohen in Cambridge, now suggests that the development of the so-called 'social brain' may be restricted in boys because for centuries it was important that males should *not* show too much sympathy for their fellows. For instance, if you are trying to kill an enemy in battle, it's not a great idea to imagine his widow or mum grieving over news of his death.

Switching off these 'social genes' in boys would produce consistent benefits. Their tendency to 'single-mindedness' would prove valuable in a warlike world. It would also provide a competitive edge in a crude industrial society where production matters more than people or pollution. It appears that twice as many of the fathers and grandfathers of autistic boys are employed as engineers than you would expect statistically. The male brain, concludes Baron-Cohen, is better constructed to think about machines than the existence, the claims or the needs of another mind.

TWO SEXES SEPARATED BY A COMMON LANGUAGE

We have to accept that John Gray's books contain a basic truth. All the psychological research shows that men and women *are* aroused by different aspects of sex, seek different rewards in sex and prefer to carry out selectively different kinds of sexual activity. And yet both sexes are stuck with the same language in which to express their contrasting desires. When trainee headhunter Geoff asked Kristine the banker at the end of their date to 'come up to his place for coffee', she was thinking about how he would kiss her while he was speculating about the colour of her underwear. While Kristine was expecting to linger over the exciting preliminaries, Geoff was plotting precise sexual positions and

SUMMARY OF SEX DIFFERENCES

Psychologist Oliver James sums up the differences thus:

women:

- Place less emphasis on sexual intercourse as a goal, are more faithful, and have fewer partners

- Fantasise less about sex, are less sexually explicit in their fantasies and focus more on the build-up than on the climax

men:

- Value physical attractiveness more highly than women do, whether it be for marriage, a date or casual sex

- Place a higher premium on sexual intercourse

- Are keener on the idea of casual sex and more indiscriminate when considering it, think more often about sex and are more unfaithful

- Fantasise about a greater variety of partners, masturbate more and are more explicit about sexual acts during fantasies

HOW TO GET MASSES OF PASSIONATE FOREPLAY

Since men and women are sometimes at odds with each other in bed there's an endless potential for confusion but the remedies can be summarised in three simple words:

communicate, communicate, communicate.

It's perfectly all right, for example, to be someone who needs masses of passionate foreplay. Perhaps it's impossible to be otherwise. If so, never apologise. Just explain, negotiate and connect. The only significant question is whether you can get what you want by word, deed or glance.

hoping, finally, that this was the girl into erotic bondage. Such can be the mental and terminological confusion between consenting members of the same species. And so the aim should be to identify these differences in order to help harmonise them.

IS THERE A GENE FOR CHATTERING?

Related to the suggestion that men are less sociable than women is the claim that they have far less aptitude for informal conversation. Women, it appears, literally like to talk more than men do. They are probably born that way. Researchers quoted by sociologist Dianne Hales in her book *Just like a Woman*, have shown that even in the womb, female foetuses exercise their jaws 30 per cent more than male ones. By the time they reach adulthood, women are uttering 23,000 words a day while the average man can only manage 12,000. Men as a whole turn out to be creatures of fewer words. This may hint at a difference of function, but men could claim to choose their words more carefully than women to avoid emotional flooding. However, women might respond that men have never understood the necessity for 'small talk' as a means of creating intimacy in personal relationships in the first place.

WHAT ABOUT 'TESTOSTERONE POISONING'?

As you may know, the hormone providing sex drive in both the sexes is called testosterone. But men usually have 20 to 40 times more of the stuff than women have. So, is this the real reason why men, for example, seem more likely to risk all they value in life – a home, marriage, career, reputation – for one illicit, risky love affair? Women, if not the nation at large, deserve an answer.

Researchers have now linked high levels of testosterone in men to both a 'higher competitive drive towards dominance' and a 'greater tendency towards sensation-seeking'. They conclude that men with average or middle levels of circulating testosterone are more prone to marital break-up than men with low levels and that men with the lowest levels of all are most satisfied by marriage and have fewest rows with their adolescent children.

Statistically speaking, these are big numbers. However, a study of 2,100 Air Force veterans by Professors Allan Mazur and Joel Michalek of Syracuse University goes even further. It shows that changes in testosterone level can indicate when divorce is likely to happen and that such changes may even cause it:

- testosterone levels are low when men first marry
- they tend to rise two years prior to a marital breakdown
- they remain unusually high until three years after the divorce

Does it start to sound familiar? The professors say these men carry their competitive attitudes into all relationships with the opposite sex. This

MEN WITH HIGH TESTOSTERONE

According to Drs Booth and Dabbs of Penn and Georgia State Universities, men with the highest concentrations of blood testosterone are 50 per cent less likely to get married in the first place. If they do marry, they are:

- 38 per cent more likely to have had extra-marital sex
- 12 per cent more likely to have hit their spouses
- 31 per cent more likely to have a temporary separation
- 43 per cent more likely to get a divorce

results in difficulty finding a spouse, and therefore not marrying. Or, once married, being unable to sustain the commitment and then divorcing. Or, if still married, having a poor quality marriage. They also show that sensation-seeking behaviour linked to testosterone levels means that men with high testosterone levels may become bored with marriage more quickly than others 'and so seek other partners thus jeopardising their domestic relationships'.

PARALLEL UNIVERSES

Even if men and women don't have conflicting hormonal systems or come from different planets, their kids learn to occupy separate social universes down here on earth. By the age of seven, boys and girls don't have best friends of the opposite sex – boys play with boys and girls with girls. And when they do play, boys tend to focus on the game while girls try to develop relationships.

In one famous experiment at the University of Denver, Colorado, 20 separate pairs of nine-year-old boys and girls were studied through a two-way mirror. In every single case the boys ignored each other 'as people', displaying no 'personal curiosity', confining their questions to technicalities of the play while the girls 'revealed over three times as much about themselves to a stranger of the same sex as did the boys'.

Afterwards, it was discovered that the girls usually liked each other a lot more while the boys stayed mutually neutral. With boys, there may be violent disagreements about interpreting the rules of a game but personal feelings are not allowed to interrupt its continuity. Girls, by contrast, are notorious for refusing to play with any friend, male or female, who has upset them. And this basic difference of approach continues until the sexes re-connect, with all such differences intact, at puberty. Puberty of course is the time when they wish to negotiate in a bigger game altogether – that of sexual attraction!

LOVE AND ATTRACTION

This difference of approach between the sexes extends to the very nature of our beliefs about sexual appeal. By and large, physical attraction hurls people together like no other force this side of an earthquake. It operates more strongly than intelligence, social skills or personality, not only on the first date but on subsequent ones too. It can operate even

YES BUT WHAT CAN YOU DO ABOUT IT?

Do not despair. What's being said is that some attractive men with high levels of sex hormones may be both sensation-seeking and competitive. They could therefore prove fascinating companions and great lovers. You would in any case expect successful people to want creative and satisfying erotic relationships. This book and its companion *How to Make Great Love to a Woman* are devoted to eliminating the boredom which puts such relationships at risk.

among children of five or six. The happiest couples are those who are most evenly matched in terms of attractiveness. It seems we tend to weigh a potential partner's attractiveness against the probability that they'd be willing to pair up with us. Put bluntly – less attractive people seek less attractive partners because they expect to be rejected by someone better-looking than themselves.

However, there is no agreement about what constitutes physical attractiveness in the first place. Men and women see things through different filters. Some of the most interesting evidence is casual – in a poll in a New York newspaper, 100 men were asked which parts of their bodies they thought were most attractive to women. One hundred women were then asked which parts of the male anatomy actually turned them on. Here are the results in order of choice:

WHAT MEN IMAGINE WOMEN ADMIRE IN MEN (%)

1 Muscular chest and shoulders (21)

2 Muscular arms (18)

3 Large penis (15)

4 Tallness (13)

5 Flat stomach (9)

6 Slimness (7)

7 Buttocks (4)

8 Hair (4)

9 Eyes (4)

10 Long legs (3)

11 Neck (2)

WHAT WOMEN REALLY ADMIRE IN MEN (%)

1 Buttocks – small and sexy (39)

2 Slimness (15)

3 Flat stomach (13)

4 Eyes (11)

5 Long legs (6)

6 Tallness (5)

7 Hair (5)

8 Neck (3)

9 Penis (2)

10 Muscular chest & shoulders (1)

11 Muscular arms (0)

As you can see, the men got it almost entirely wrong. The bewildering difference between the two sets of answers provides a big clue to the way men see themselves sexually. Women would certainly profit by understanding the discrepancy. We can also see which aspects of body image make men feel the most vulnerable. The fundamental fallacy is that *men obviously expect women to admire them for the qualities that will impress other men* – big muscles and large genitals. If anything, it's *men* who suffer from penis envy, an organ which incidentally only two per cent of women felt was worth a mention. As a rule of thumb, therefore, you might find it useful to tell your man how much you admire his manly biceps, triceps and remarkable phallus rather than his pert, petite derrière.

HOW YOU ARE LIKELY TO APPEAL TO YOUR MAN

More scientific evidence comes from studies exploring the popular assumption that males can be classified by their tastes as 'breast, bottom or leg men'. Researchers at the University of Illinois discovered interesting links with personality types, at least in the USA. They say:

breasts:
- Men who react most strongly to large busts are likely to consume soft pornography, smoke a lot, date frequently and be keen on sport.
- Men who like small breasts drink little, are more likely to be involved in religion and display more depressive and submissive characteristics.

bottoms:
- Men who like large bottoms tend to be obsessive, passive, guilt-prone and to support strong government.
- Men who prefer small bottoms are persistent in their work and devoid of interest in macho activities like sport.

legs:
- Men who like large legs usually abstain from alcohol, are more self-abasing, socially inhibited and under-motivated.
- Men who want partners with 'petite' legs are likely to be more sociable, exhibitionistic, nurturing and more extrovert.

In general, say the researchers, men who like large figures are those who need their lives to succeed materially and publicly. Men who want smaller women are more introverted and likely to be self-sufficient. Now this evidence isn't likely to guide you when choosing or evaluating a man. But it *is* worth considering how the attraction system within the male psyche tends to operate. 'The preferences of men for different types of female figure are linked with their general personality and life style,' says psychologist Dr Glenn Wilson summarising the findings. Other research at the University of Oxford confirms the general suggestion that sporty extroverts go for busty girls and submissive introverts prefer their women to be more 'elfin'.

What use is this to you? We're certainly not suggesting that you diet or in any way try to alter your appearance. What we do think is useful

CASE HISTORY

Henry, a 29-year-old telecoms manager, is an example of this extrovert sporty type. On the surface, life with Henry was a blast. He was always up-to-date with the latest Internet jokes, which he would tell at the least appropriate moments. His parties were legendary, his support for the home-town football team extreme. He was not present at the birth of his first child, because his side was playing an important home fixture. A year before, he had fallen foul of company sexual harassment rules by complimenting his secretary on her brassiere, saying he was happy to see it 'fighting a losing battle to keep her under control'. It was the sort of remark, common enough in the past, which people find unacceptable today.

His relationship to his wife Ruthie had taken a turn for the worse with the birth of their daughter, Patricia. Ruthie was wounded by Henry's apparent indifference on the big day. Henry was disconcerted to find himself no longer the centre of attention in Ruthie's life. They had arguments about her not wanting to resume sex after the birth. Then, when they did plan an evening's lovemaking, Henry found himself to be impotent, and blamed everyone but himself for the problem. He even became seriously irrational and started quizzing Ruthie about her lovers prior to marriage – wanting to know how they touched and what sexual activities took place. The relationship hit rock bottom (and this was when Ruthie sought out therapy) when Henry forced Ruthie to drive 100 miles to a beach in the middle of the night where she had once made love with a special boyfriend nine years earlier. Henry tried to dig up the spot in the sand and 'throw it away'.

Moral: don't mistake the packaging for a man's real sexual confidence. Advertising isn't truth. Look beneath the surface.

is to look at the motivation behind those types of men. It could be valuable to know that the classifications conceal some fascinating internal contradictions.

Extrovert sporty men, for example, may feel internally less strong and even inferior. Hence their attention-seeking behaviour. They will be attracted to women whose nubile bodies 'make a public statement on their behalf'. Their message to other men could be roughly translated as 'envy me!' And naturally, as partners, men of this sort may prove jealous, demanding and prone to crisis when age or disillusion take their toll. So we would suggest that you look out for contradictory reasons for your male's attitudes towards life.

THE SECRETS OF SEXUAL FANTASY

We said earlier that men have a different fantasy process from women. Whereas women fantasise at least partly about their regular partners, focussing on the 'journey' not the 'arrival', men tend to fantasise about almost anyone they meet on the way, with the emphasis on novelty and a big climax. According to most surveys, the biggest recorded difference between men and women is 'making love in a romantic setting' which 15 per cent of women do in fantasies compared to only four per cent of men. About 10 per cent of women think about 'passionately kissing their partners' whereas none of the men seemed to let this cross their minds. Four times as many women as men dream about cunnilingus. Eight times as many men as women dream about 'being promiscuous' and 'seducing an innocent'. When it comes to kinky fantasies about group sex, whipping and bondage, men always outscored the women, although the question of boastfulness versus lying is one to ponder.

HOW MANY TIMES A DAY DO MEN THINK ABOUT SEX?

Men and women seem to fantasise for roughly equal amounts of time. It is not true that 'men are thinking about sex every five minutes whereas women only think about it when they fall in love'. Research that maps human eye movements in men and women demonstrates that both sexes, when given an opportunity to meet new and attractive people, check them out in all the obvious and traditional places – chests, breasts, buttocks and genitals. Content, in fact, turns out to be the principal sexual difference. Glenn Wilson theorises that in men fantasies happen

FANTASIES

Male sexual fantasies can be grouped into predictable clusters.

Men are especially excited by:

- Women who find them irresistible
- Women who are submissive
- Women who are dominant
- Women in a harem
- The lesbian ménage-à-trois
- The stranger who offers sex with no questions asked
- The woman who offers oral sex
- The woman who wants to sit on a man's face
- The woman in skimpy underwear
- The big-breasted Miss World-winner offering sex
- The older 'Mrs Robinson' figure who offers sex
- The exhibitionist 'Sharon Stone' figure who lets men look up her skirt
- The 'Demi Moore' boss who demands sex from employees
- The dizzy secretary who offers sex under her desk

And so on.

Notice that typical male sexual fantasies do not include a woman swearing eternal faithful love in an undying marital union. Men's erotic dreams are most frequently about power, ego and control. Accordingly, there's a conflict between the sexual and social cultures men inhabit and this can lead to stresses and tensions in intimate relationships. Of course, neither sex can 'choose' the fantasies that it finds more exciting and men have been conditioned over thousands of years to include these competitive genetic traits.

The fact that society today needs less, not more, aggressive male sexuality cannot be readily instilled into our minds. At one level, both sexes must learn to accept things the way they are and treat male sexuality as a system to be enjoyed within its own limits!

when their sex drive is not totally fulfilled, whereas women seem to have more fantasies when their sex life is going well.

THREE CLASSIC MALE FANTASY SCENARIOS

1 **Power trip:** 'I imagine being the mayor of a small town filled with nude girls from 20 to 24. I like to take walks and pick out the best-looking one that day, and she engages in intercourse with me. All the women have sex with me any time I want.'

2 **Visual feast:** 'I'd like to step back during intercourse and watch myself in a mirror while my girlfriend fellates me. Unfortunately this remains a fantasy because I've had difficulty in persuading my dates to comply with this preference.'

3 **Primal unclothing:** 'When I was 11, I used to think about one of my female friends and imagine us going off into the woods near the school by ourselves and taking off all our clothes. I would then touch her all over her body especially in her genital area. She would take off her underwear, exposing her body, and then take off my clothes. Today, I think about a grown-up girl who takes off her clothes. I especially think about her unsnapping her bra. I can see her exposing her breasts and thighs. I also think about her unzipping my pants to expose my penis.' (Quoted: Glenn Wilson, *The Secrets of Sexual Fantasy*, Dent.)

WHAT TURNS MEN ON

So what does turn men on when they let their imaginations roam?

Male fantasy involves:
- Their partner's attractions
- Actually having sex
- Female subjects who are nearly always 'willing' and compliant
- Many different women (who are mostly anonymous)
- Sexual situations very like those enjoyed during adolescence
- Little personal attachment or interpersonal involvement with the women featured in the fantasies

CONCLUSION

So what can you do with all this? When thinking about how to make love to a man, it is obviously wise to consider both similarities and differences. Boys can never 'turn into their mums' because they have to behave, sound and dress in a male style. By virtue of growing up male they cannot retain purely female thought processes. Unlike girls, boys have to make an emotional journey away from their mother and toward their father. In behaviour and development, girls have the choice of remaining closer to their mothers. Around the age of five, differences begin to excite suspicion and ridicule. Traditionally, boys have made fun of menstruation because it is alien to their experience. Girls rarely understand why men are so concerned about the length and girth of the penis. (It isn't really because they want to be hung like horses, they want more status). Later on, when hormones begin to bombard adolescent bodies, the picture changes. Suddenly this joint incomprehension becomes alluring.

But there's more to it than that. These days, the sexes are taking on each other's characteristics. Many 12-year-old girls now play soccer. More and more boys are becoming enthusiastic about cooking. The need in a modern relationship for overlap of function and talent affects us all. And in the bedroom (or bathroom or back seat of car or park bench), women are coming to understand that men are not innately more aggressive and dominant – that was just a label from history. Men are increasingly keen on finding a soulmate. But a soulmate is the woman who accepts and enjoys a man's masculine enthusiasms, because she shares many of them while retaining her essential femininity.

Where sex differences still remain is in the understanding of each other's systems. The average woman needs to know that the average man needs far more sexual novelty and emotional routine than she does. If the goal for both men and women is improved intimacy (plus great sex), then the means to get there is by appreciating each other's peculiarities of character and unique strengths. This means no more taking each other for granted. No instant assumption that what he likes, you will like. No more beliefs that all men are the same and will possess the same sexual approach. Every male is subtly different from the next. Just like you women!

With this blow-by-blow account of male sexual preference under your belt, let's look now at your first serious love affair, the subject of the next chapter. Just what are the best ways to persuade a chap that he's discovered the love of his life? Read on.

SUMMARY

❦ Men live on your planet

❦ They initially and instinctively respond to emotional problems with avoidance

❦ Open conflict makes them anxious

❦ They are less verbally able to defend themselves

❦ Judged by life expectancy, they seek out more novelty and excitement than is good for them

❦ Men are insecure about their physical appearance and sexual performance

❦ They try to sense – usually with their eyes – the way in which the world regards and judges them

2

THE beginnings OF LOVE

In many ways, the following applies to a love affair whether you are nineteen or 90. But when you first fall in love with a young man of 18–30, be aware that he has only just emerged from the highly competitive world of telling lies to his friends about his sexual performance and experience. A lot of masculine identity rests on the slippery slope of sexual success. Sexually, men hit their peak around 20 – unlike women, who are probably most responsive and receptive at around 30. A massive eightfold rise in sex hormones at 13 or 14 means your beau is now thinking about sex every day. But it's triple-think. First, he craves a passionate union with you. Second, he fancies the same with almost every other woman. Third, he's a natural spin doctor – eager to impress peers and partners alike with his virility stories. So making love to him at this stage needs to be done with a firm sense of separating the wood from the trees and hype from reality. Lots of physical reassurance is essential – so be prepared to spend hours in the nude.

CASE HISTORY

When Suzanne, the University French and Spanish coach, started teaching modern languages to Raymond the 22-year-old, she didn't plan to fall in love. There was the little matter of a 20-year age gap. But her marriage had been punctuated by a humiliating series of infidelities on the part of her husband, the Professor of Engineering. This time, she felt compelled to retaliate. Her revenge did not run smoothly:

'Raymond was very inexperienced and I was worried about his discretion. I'd lots to lose and he was quite overcome by the fact that an older woman was showing such interest in him. It made him bumptious – even cocky. I had to say "Slow down" to him more than once, and I even once remarked "You have never before made love to a woman who has had children, have you?" – which didn't help his confidence. In the end, I had to show him where I needed him to touch me and which sexual positions brought me to orgasm. However, I loved having this man and I don't think he really minded.'

Remember that until a man has sexually 'done everything' at least once, he's likely to remain a bit of a spectator at his own pleasure. By that I mean that he will be on the outside of the experience, not specially relaxed and his observational brain will be working overtime. He may also pretend that he already knows what he's doing while at the same time desperately copying the moves you make, trying to second-guess what you want.

When your lover is this inexperienced, it pays to be reassuring. I don't mean you should accept insensitivity. But if he pretends to know your body better than you do, or handles you as roughly as he would himself, or tries to put his legs outside yours when it's wiser to adopt a less ambitious posture, guide him. Express your desire encouragingly – 'I love it when you do X' – rather than – 'Not that way, silly!' If his erection fails or the climax is premature, don't turn it into a drama or a crisis. Just carry on kissing. There's almost certainly nothing physically wrong with him, so it's best to let caresses move elsewhere till *you're* satisfied. Young men can bounce back.

THE DATING GAME

Recently, *Cosmopolitan* published Phillip Hodson's guide to love, sex and relationships contrasting the way we date now with the way things used to be even a few years ago:

'**Today**: *boy meets girl. After three weeks, they find the time to go out to dinner. They discuss job stress. They eat the food of love – exotic mushrooms, wild strawberries – but it makes no impression on them. They think that the candlelight is some sort of remedy for tired eyes. She's frazzled and didn't bother to 'fix' her appearance. He's dyspeptic from the shouting match he had with his account manager. They do like each other. They think, in the abstract, about their respective attractions. They could get a wonderful romance together if God gave them six months off on a desert island. But after coffee (decaffeinated) they take their separate transport home. He doesn't dream of making a pass – nobody does in the middle of the week. She wouldn't say yes if he did. She'll be asleep before her heads hits the pillow. The alarm is set for 6.30 and she's got to stay focused.*

Fifteen years ago: boy met girl. They agreed to a date later that day. They knocked off work at 4.30, dashed home, primped and preened. He collected her by car to cut off her escape at the end of the evening. The romantic meal would be carefully chosen to fill her stomach with spice and her veins with a measure of pure alcohol. Both would be playing a game, with her running just fast enough to let him catch her if she wanted him to. The meal was foreplay and the only major decision was timing – would they do it on the first date, the second or third? Whatever was decided, the evening was just an episode in that long-running saga of Let's Make Love. And both were keen'.

MEN WHO FEEL THE DATING STRAIN

There are other reasons besides physical ones for men's intermittent sexual confidence. Ralph, a 24-year-old publishing executive, on his third bottle of Becks, complains: 'It's a common male bleat I know, but why do men still have to do all the work? Why are men always expected to cross the dance floor and approach the woman? Why aren't women more pro-active? In my perfect world, I would sit in a club and the woman would come and talk to me and I'd never have to risk falling flat on my face again. It's a kind of male fantasy of course, but that's what women expect men to do all the time'.

HOW DO YOU NEGOTIATE WITH A NEW LOVER?

In our seven day a week, 24-hour a day workaholic world, there are no longer clear rules of sexual engagement. The following are all acceptable gambits:

- 'Could I spend the night with you and you just hold me in your arms?' *(36-year-old Jane to 27-year-old Peter).*

- 'I'm sorry, I won't sleep with you because you're leaving the country in two months' time.' *(24-year-old Lydia to 31-year-old Greg).*

- 'Will you come home and fuck me?' *(30-year-old Donna to 29-year-old Chris at a party).*

- 'Let's take the sex side really slowly because it's worth enjoying and getting right.' *(24-year-old Sheena to 29-year-old George).*

Traditionally, men are the asking sex. They ask for dates and in most societies they are still expected to take the lead sexually. So men are inevitably the sex which invites rejection. At the heart of male sexuality, therefore, is a kind of mating masochism. In order to be fulfilled, a man must expose himself to the critical scrutiny and potential damnation of the woman he desires. His life is governed by her one-sided power of veto. And the world today still expects him to take most of it on the chin.

Amazingly, there seems to be at least one good woman for every good man but at a price in male ego and pride. All of us pay this entrance fee at the standard rate. But, for men who are unlucky, unattractive, inept or shy, the rate is more like extortion. After an accumulation of such rejection, anyone would become defensive and disposed to throw himself into that river of oblivion known as denial. Men may say 'rejection doesn't hurt'. (It's interesting that Ralph uses a word like 'bleat' as if men were as feeble as sheep.) But we all know that this is false. Men, as a sex, cut themselves off from feelings, then over-compensate. As we walked into the bank the other day, the man in front went up to the female cashier and boomed: 'Are you available? That's what I want to know from all the young women I meet.' This was crass and sexist but made us think that hidden in this tired old chat was a desperate little plea: 'Please tell me you might somewhere find me interesting'. In the hearts of men there's a lot of pathetic self-advertising.

ARE YOU BOTH INTERESTED?

So most men will be grateful if you give clearer signals about your initial level of interest. This is firstly about the type of *eye contact* you use. Once you have noticed a man whom you fancy across a crowded room, the chances are that your eyes will meet his and linger just slightly longer than they would normally. It's important that he 'sees you seeing him' before you glance away. Then you do it again. If both parties keep on looking, there's a good chance that he's willing to enter into a conversation. However, if he frowns or looks irritated, don't bother. The game is traditionally one where the male is supposed to reveal slightly more interest – but all surveys show that men like it when women also reinforce the first move.

READING A MAN'S SEXUAL SIGNALS

A man is also likely to be interested in you sexually when he:

- Touches your arm or back during conversations
- Holds his body at right angles to yours, or stands in front with one leg advanced towards you
- Leans 'into' you while standing
- Puts his hands on his neck or raises his arms
- Plays with his collar or neckline, or fidgets with a button
- Licks his lips
- Opens his eyes very wide
- Uncrosses his legs while seated opposite to you

But be sensible. Sometimes people cross their legs because they want to go to the bathroom, not keep you at bay!

YOUR SEXUAL SCENT

Pheromones are the chemicals that help men decide whether or not to fancy you. Studies show that you are most attractive to a man when you are ovulating – in other words, when you are at the peak of your fertility. Apparently, men and women have developed a mechanism that allows them literally to sniff out when a woman is most ripe for getting with child (a move that made good evolutionary sense for our cave-dwelling ancestors, as it does for all primates). Noses can detect the sensual secrets of pheromones, which are themselves triggered by critical levels of female sex hormones, above all oestrogen. This, of course, is present at its highest levels during ovulation.

ADRENALINE RUSH

Lured like a moth to the flame by the heady scent of pheromones, the amorous male is further aroused by the visual stimuli that you offer at the time of ovulation. These include dilated pupils and a general 'glow' and are the work of an intriguing chemical known as PEA, or phenylethylamine. Already hot with lust, the man's fires are stoked still further by the release of a blast of adrenaline (which makes him giddy).

More hormones spark. His testosterone levels rise, making him more adventurous and frisky, while your elevated oestrogen increases potential receptivity to his advances. Brain neurotransmitters get in on the action. Levels of serotonin drop, relaxing inhibitions and generally improving mood, while dopamine hits the bloodstream, intensifying sexual desire. It's at this stage that PEA takes over. Its effects account for many of the classic sensations of falling in love, including butterflies in the tummy, breathlessness, rapid pulse, dry mouth, low appetite, excitement and general euphoria, and the radiant glow of infatuation. It comes as no surprise to learn that PEA is related to the amphetamines. PEA also occurs naturally in chocolate and roses.

So look at yourself and look at him. Does he appear to be flushed with adrenaline? If not, it's simple. Let him smell you. Raise an arm in his direction. Use any opportunity to get close enough for him to collect your scent. Then, if you catch a glance of yourself in the mirror, you may notice that your face is shining. And possibly your eyes are sparkling? If so, we suggest you are showing strong signs of romantic interest. If not, and you'd like to grow more responsive, see if you can catch a hint of his scent – the most erotic chemicals are found in unfashionable places – the chest, even the armpit of love, but obviously use your common sense. An arousing male aroma is one thing – bad odour another.

PACING

Once you've broken the ice, remember that the besetting sin of most male teens and 20-somethings is haste. This is nervousness rather than a true desire to break the world land-speed record for sexual intercourse. Make a conscious effort to get him to savour, linger and dally. All acts of love are a mixture of one person finding out what they want and showing the other how to deliver. If you really want to feel safe and comfortable, begin your physical relationship by holding hands. There's nothing wrong in taking this initiative, nor any threat in the gesture itself. You can quickly tell if it feels comfortable for both, and if you do it in the dark at the movies, in the car, on the couch or somewhere else classically intimate, this old-fashioned act can bring considerable sexual closeness before any real bridges have been crossed. So play with his arm, wrist, fingers or palm – when you want. Men carry this handy item of equipment round with them all the time.

LAY LINES

We also think it helps if you can appreciate the lie of the sexual 'lay lines'. This should of course read LEY lines. You've heard of those mysterious lines possessing magical properties, which are supposed to run through the earth between major features of the landscape. Well, there are also sexual 'ley' lines running throughout the human body between features such as his brain and genitals. Curiously, no one seems to know much about them, so you've got your hands on a world erotic exclusive.

What's involved? Well, it's not acupuncture, since the connections are focused on gratification rather than healing. It's not quite reflexology since we're not talking pressure points. It's certainly not softball – racing from first base to fourth base in order to 'score'. What you're trying to do is trace those areas of skin where meridian nerves that send impulses to the spinal sex centre rise closest to the surface. We'll say that again – you want to touch your man erotically where science suggests

HOW TO MAKE A FOREARM COME IN THE CINEMA

The Jesuits used to say 'Give me a child up to the age of seven and I'll make him a Catholic for life'. We say 'Obtain unrestricted access to your man's forearm at the local multiplex for 40 minutes and we guarantee he'll want to see you again and *mean* it'.

Sitting on his right, holding his right hand in your left with your elbows on the arm-rest, stick your popcorn on the floor and gaze deeply at the screen. Casually unbutton his shirt sleeve with your free right hand till he's naked to the elbow. Now imagine a line starting at the mid-point of the base of his palm where the blue veins gather and proceeding for about nine inches along the tendon of the forearm.

Clasping his hand firmly in yours to prevent wriggling, gently trace an insistent pattern with a couple of fingernails along the underarm from wrist to elbow and back again. It's essential to have long but manicured nails like a classical guitar player and keep the touches varied, persistent, measured but not 'tickly'. The golden rule is never to hurry. If you follow the prescribed route and keep in the groove, you should notice after a few minutes that your partner begins to squirm ever so slightly in his seat, as if this ley line were linked directly to his pelvis. In fact, it terminates in his spinal sex centre and penis, which is why he can't keep still.

To test progress, cease your action in mid-stroke and see whether there's a gasp. If he re-submits his arm for attention, you're doing quite well.

he's least defended. Imagine using different ley lines at different stages of your new relationship. On a first date, you might want to start by charming an arm.

THE NECK

Ley lines are particularly concentrated in the neck area. As the body narrows at this point, the wiring gets packed tight round the vertebral column. We all know that the earlobes are specially sexy but even more sensual lines can be discovered down the sides of the neck from a point half an inch behind and below the ears to the collar-bone cavities. These cervical tracks are easily touched by hands or lips. So on or after the first date, make sure your lips and tongue give feather-like touches to these parts. You'll be able to tell when it's effective – he'll suffer anything from local tingling to all-over shivers of delight.

THE SPINAL TAP

By the third or fourth date, your relationship may be intimate but not entirely free-and-easy so it's often a good idea to suggest a bit of massage. This allows everyone to retain their underwear and dignity. At the same time, you only need to gain moderate access to the spine to command one of the body's busiest sexual motorways. Of course the secret is *not* to restrict yourself to an ordinary massage. Silly. Rather, with an ultra slow-moving tongue-tip, attempt to resurface his skin from waist to skull following the natural line of the spine. All you do is lick. To be delectable, the touch must be barely detectable. Imagine you can see the tiny baby hairs peeping up from the dorsal skin. It's these you have to lift and titivate. Use a little saliva and make progress by milli-metres not inches. It should take at least one minute to run from waist-line to hairline. When you touch the neck, expect an almighty whoosh of breath from somewhere beneath you as the nerve sends sensation all the way from the neck to the area of skin near the penis (the perineum). Who said you can't be in three places at the same time? Then repeat again from the midriff.

LEGWORK

Neural pathways connect the whole body to the sex centres of the spine and the brain for one very good reason. The purpose of our species is reproduction and you never know when a passing reproducer is going to put a hand on your knee. Or better still, on the inside or outside leg where some major nerves can be accessed. These lie along the sides of the legs from just above the ankle to just before the knee, and again from just after the knee to the highly sensitive hollow of the buttocks. Most responsive, of course, are the inner thighs where if your partner is unsure whether they are ready to go all the way, a successful case can usually be made if you stroke the ley lines up to but not beyond the perineal divide. Start two inches up from the inside knee to the scrotum and go no further. They say this is what happens in massage parlours. If you want your man to ask for 'extras', make sure your touches fall tantalisingly short of his testes.

BUTTOCKS AREN'T BAD

As your relationship matures, you will begin to know your partner's principal ley lines from head to toe. When all these networks have been explored, we personally would plump for the buttocks – about two inches either side of the global points north-south – where a teasing caress can not only cause instant reaction, it will make him sick with longing. The most sensitive parts of the body are sometimes the least visited and let's face it, his buttocks mainly get sat upon. Yet their primary nerves are deeply attached to the stomach, the pc (pubococcygeal) muscles controlling the 'orgasmic platform' of the prostate as well as his adrenal glands. So, if you've ever wanted to mix adrenaline with ecstasy, try a flanking manoeuvre.

STEALING KISSES

Most men like being kissed (although some people of both sexes remain kissophobic). Again, you need to realise that men often regard the act of kissing in terms of progress towards acts of sexual intercourse whereas many women just like kissing. Not for nothing do American males employ a baseball metaphor – running around the bases until they reach the goal of 'home' and score – to measure their sexual progress. Sometimes they need help to understand that kissing can be fun even when it goes no further than first base – the kissing base.

LUSCIOUS LIPWORK

If you want to kiss your man into distraction, then the following are nearly always bound to work:

- Dark red lipstick:
  Men are usually visually aroused. Colours that remind them of a full sex blush or flush are known to work best.

- Lipgloss, which perhaps suggests the sheen of sweat on a body that is in heat.

- A mixture of teasing gentle lip caresses intermixed with sudden full-pressure surges of eat-my-tonsils desire and the odd nippy bite. Blood should only be drawn by the serious.

- A bold intruding tongue helps to break down mental barriers to further intimacy and familiarity.

- Serious groans of passion that men will probably assume relate to their own sex appeal.

MANAGING A NAKED YOUNG MAN

Don't be surprised by anything you find. There can be a mix of sexual ignorance and sophistication. Some young men will tremble all over whenever you touch them. Others will be coarse and greedy. Others will be over-keen to please you. Some men are 'born givers' and believe that sex is what men do to women. Still others are sexually selfish and expect women to give sex to them.

Most like to avoid courtship's agonies of ambiguity. What attracted males to the otherwise unpleasant character of 'Mrs Robinson' in the movie *The Graduate* was her cut-and-dried offer: 'Benjamin, do you want to make love to me?' It is the most enormous relief for a man to have his doubts removed at the beginning of any new encounter. In fact, that particular film where Anne Bancroft plays a sex symbol in her 40s demonstrates the extent of young male anxiety. If his sexual doubt is the question, here are the answers:

- A mature woman climbs on a bar stool and opens her legs beneath a short skirt in a gesture of obvious invitation.
- She reinforces this with a clear verbal invitation to intercourse.
- She promises to give a kind of operational sex education to the virginal boy.
- She swears (perhaps hastily) there will be no strings of any kind.
- She implies great sexual passion is really possible free of emotional involvement.

REFLECTION

You will not find the average teenage student being able to sustain intercourse beyond about ten to 15 minutes at most. Moreover, his direction of thrusting will probably seem remiss. From a man's viewpoint, the thrust itself provides the excitement and pleasure. The penile angle – so important to make contact with your clitoris or G-spot – is of no special interest to him. The average male will also have masturbated in a series of continuously speeded up strokes towards climax rather than by using a stop-start process and this will condition his attitude towards the 'proper' way to make love. So bear this in mind, when you want to give a good time. And if you want to get a good time, make sure foreplay is prolonged.

LOVE POSITIONS THAT WORK FOR MEN

Positions for sexual intercourse are very much a matter of choice and taste. For instance, two ballet dancers could obviously deploy more athletic postures than a husband with his heavily pregnant wife can. But sex is not just about choreography. It's also about being comfortable with your sexual personality. Everyone has a preferred style of love-making and each couple will naturally prefer some positions to others. These will probably be the ones that are best adapted to they way your two bodies fit. And yet, if sex does get stuck in a routine, new positions can add unexpected pleasure and delight. Some positions help and others hinder orgasm by the man – so checking on the options is sometimes essential. But don't consider sex as taking place in one fixed position – each can be varied and develop into the next as the mood develops and sex continues in a variety of simple tableaux.

MAN ON TOP

❦ Missionary with his legs inside hers. Very traditional because very comfortable. Good for the heavily-built. Face-to-face is highly personal and friendly. It also permits easy kissing of lips and breasts. Gratifying for men who feel the need to be in charge. Allows the woman to stroke his buttocks and back. The man can lean forward to press the front of his penis onto her clitoris. Either sex can slip a finger down between the bodies to give the necessary attention to her clitoris but this sometimes feels awkward causing wrist-ache. Can become …

❦ Missionary with her legs closed and his now on the outside. This is an excellent position to give her a breather from deep penetration while switching to clitoral focus. Excellent for him if he needs extra pressure on his penis (and testicles) to trip him into climax. Won't work for men with more modest penile proportions, nor when the woman has very wide hips compared to the male. Can vary into …

❦ Missionary with him now putting his legs back inside hers then moving her legs under his arms and raising her pelvis off the bed. Only attempt if you can tolerate the deeper penetration. The result again partly depends on penis size, so use common sense. If deeper penetration is bliss, or if you are trying to reach the G-spot, then your legs can be draped over his shoulders and you can bend back almost double on the bed. Ask him to use care with his forward thrusts in reaching your G-spot but let him know when he is on target (men like military metaphors). The man should half-withdraw his penis then start pressing quite hard with the tip against the firmness of the pubic bone (if necessary by pressing his body downwards). Explain he may have to move around a little bit until he strikes the spot, but with a bit of luck you will suddenly want to say something to him along the lines of 'Mmmm … don't move!' At this point, hold the pressure and see if you can reach the most dramatic climax without any further in-out thrusts. You could add: 'Just there … don't move … oh yessss … keep still … oh it's like the world's spinning, it's unbearable, I want it to go on forever'. A common variant of this position is to raise just one of your legs so the vagina is even more exposed and your clitoris more likely to be stimulated by the penile shaft. From this posture, it's relatively easy to switch to …

🐝 Doggy fashion, with woman face down and the man's legs still inside hers (or outside as preferred). The move from missionary to doggy can be achieved without his penis leaving the vagina by a rotary manoeuvre or you can briefly break-off and re-insert.
He can now kiss your highly sensuous neck, while you can easily reach your clitoris yourself. His weight is distributed across your body so the energy drain is minimal. Your bottom feels wonderful under his abdomen. This can rapidly change into…

🐝 Doggy fashion with both partners kneeling but her hands on the floor. This position works best if his upper leg bone is roughly the right length to bring his penis to exactly the same height as your vagina. The thrusts can be rapid and he can grasp handfuls of breasts or reach round to both vulva and clitoris. He can also stroke your buttocks at will or grasp your hair to pull you harder onto his penis with a symbolic gesture of control. Both parties can regulate the speed of thrusting but you do need to co-ordinate.
If you don't meet his upstroke, but move away instead, the result is missed friction or frustration rather than pleasure. The position easily moves into …

🐝 Doggy fashion with her arms and chin on the floor. Now you can again feel penile pressure on the clitoris but less on the G-spot.
He has the visual delight of seeing your bottom fully spread and presented for his inspection and attention. It is a wanton posture, full of animal intent. If G-spot attention is required, this position easily transforms into …

🐝 Doggy fashion with him half standing. All the man does is raise himself on his legs supporting his weight by placing hands on your hips and thrusting downwards. This can feel a little strained and you need to be fit enough to hold the body weight but the feeling for the man is one of highly-sexual possession.

WOMAN ON TOP

❣ Missionary with you straddling him or your legs lying on top of his. This has all the pluses and minuses as when the man is on top except that now you will be doing the work. Some men find this the best position when worried about impotence or being only 'semi-hard'. They can grip the base of the penis by hand while the woman lowers herself onto the erection and so reduce performance anxiety. This position easily changes into …

❣ The woman raises up her legs and kneels astride or even squats on the man's erection. Stimulation is increased by rocking or pumping vigorously or, in the kneeling variant, by sliding enthusiastically forwards and backwards. Lovely sensation for him in particular as the whole of your perineal region, moistly lubricated, slithers across his genital zone. In the squatting variant, it's easy to change the position to …

❣ Face to face sitting up with your legs over his. This is the 'cuddle' position allowing maximum hugging and kissing. The position is great for reaching down to add finger-tip spice to what's happening with the genitals. Now it's simplicity itself to roll into …

SIDE BY SIDE POSITIONS

Either adopt the 'spoon' position, with the man thrusting from behind while holding you with an arm wrapped across your chest and caressing your breasts. Or, you should raise your lower leg so you can fit together like a pair of scissors. Or, he should enter you at right angles with your bodies in a cross-shape. This position will suddenly permit sharp and different sensations to both partners – the man should be wary of coming before he is ready as the penis is gripped from above and below by the vaginal lips.

None of the above positions is difficult, complicated or requires excess physical exertion. They can all be enjoyed in a natural sequence of moves allowing both partners to maximize their erotic pleasure.

ADVANCED LOVEMAKING POSITIONS

These are included here for the sake of completeness. Perhaps you wouldn't be attempting these with a relatively inexperienced younger lover. The only sense in which these positions can be called 'advanced' is that they require an extra degree of strength or agility which some couples will not possess. Nor does 'advanced' imply that other, common positions are ordinary or second best.

- Standing up – is included because you do need to carry a fair amount of body weight in the upstroke whether the man or woman is doing the work. The position is highly erotic whether face to face or from behind because it has a raw physicality or impatience about it. Lovers of the outdoors will know this position. Also favoured by those carried away on a date.

- Doggy style but with the man lying on his back, the woman also lying back, your feet supporting your weight on the ground either side of his thighs. The beauty of this energetic posture is the way the man feels taken over by the woman while he can still grasp her breasts from below. For you, the main advantage is the intense G-spot pressure you can apply simply by leaning further back against his penile head.

- The wheelbarrow with him standing while entering you from behind. He supports your body weight with arms linked beneath your tummy (or with your elbows resting on a chair) while you lock your feet behind his back. Sounds difficult but is actually relatively simple provided you are fairly supple. Some people wonder what the fuss is all about with this position; others say you have to try it to find out.

We feel that it is important to say, having offered you this extensive list of gymnastic positions, that swinging from the banisters is not everything. Once you know such physical options are available to you, it's probably best to put the list to the back of your mind and only use it if you feel that you need a bit of inspiration. Otherwise, do what comes naturally – enjoy the spontaneous. Our list is for reference – as you consider the longer-term joys of the next chapter on Settling Down.

Passionately SETTLING DOWN

3

'My heart sinks when I meet a couple joined at the hip. You know the sort I mean – they've never had a cross word in years and he turns to her and says "Do I have salt on my potatoes?" I think it's a recipe for a coma' – Rivka Pomson, Therapist

Marriage is no guaranteed aphrodisiac and nor is cohabitation. You will find subtle but inevitable changes in a loving sexual relationship over the first few years. Probably, you will be forced to spend more nights apart and more days building your career. Gradually, you may feel that it's been too much time since your were alone together and at peace. Parents and children may intrude as much as work does. Finding a place to live can be tough. Life quality may not seem what it was. In effect, you are managing the difficult transition from lovers to partners. What you don't want is to sacrifice the deeper rewards of passion along the way. Getting the balance right is hard. So no apologies from us for looking at the negative pressures first. If you want your erotic intimacy to survive, the paradox to face is the absolute need to retain a separate identity. Contrary to the cliché, good relationships are not about merging your personalities but retaining an interesting and attractive independent self. In order to keep the spice, you need a life.

PATTERNS TO AVOID

We once met a couple who were never out of each other's sight. Janet and Roger went to the bathroom together, ate together, shopped together, saw the dentist and even her gynaecologist together. They dressed in the same, dim greens and browns. They always slept in the same bed like Sir Paul and the late Linda McCartney. Thinking each other's thoughts, ending each other's sentences – they believed divorce was a dirty word and the product of a sick society. They'd drawn up a suicide pact to die together if one of them should fall fatally ill. Now the big question is do you envy them or hate them?

Psychologists claim that we divide fifty-fifty. Pushed to the limit, half the population suspect that hell is living alone, the rest think hell is being surrounded by others. But couples pay a high price if they think that they can survive in splendid isolation forever. The church isn't a lot of help: 'When you make the two one, and make the inside like the outside, and the outside like the inside, and the upper side like the under side, and in such a way that you make the man with the woman a single one … then you will go into the Kingdom' (according to St Thomas).

So here are ten reasons why you need to think hard before you turn your long-term partner into some sort of Siamese twin. What we're really saying is that it's a bad idea to put all your eggs in one basket and then do nothing but watch the basket!

1 First, and obviously, there's an enormous danger that when a crisis happens – as inevitably it does – you will need other people to get you through the night. If your only friend on the planet is your partner for life and he has just decided the grass is greener with the woman he met on the Internet, you will find yourself up in the air without a parachute and lacking someone to help you see things in perspective. If you survive, you land in a pit of depression. It's then that you depend on friends. 'Friends are the family of our own invention,' says agony aunt Irma Kurtz, 'and women simply cannot live without them.'

2 The cult of 'togetherness' is under fire even from conservative traditionalists: 'Everyone needs a certain amount of privacy, which is why middle-class men used to have studies and working-class chaps had garden sheds or allotments. The current vogue for togetherness is disastrous and why many marriages break up' (*Daily Mail*). In a recent episode of a US sitcom, the wife of the heroine's former boyfriend says: 'I thought marriage meant never having any secrets from each other' to be told: 'No, I promised to respect my other friends' confidences too'.

3 If tradition insists that wives should blend into husbands like flour into a cake you also have to decide who gets the bigger cut. It's a sixties recipe revisited: 'When two are made one, the important question is Which One?' Do you really move house and follow your husband because he's been seconded to Seattle for two years or do you stay in blissful Gloucestershire/Scotland/Hyde Park Gardens and get him to help you with your Computer Software and Catering Business? The choice is for *both* of you. And he needs you to be strong enough to put your viewpoint forward.

4 At a deeper level, says North London-based psychotherapist Rivka Pomson, we get trapped by rituals: 'There's a tradition that men should take the lead in everything from marriage to waltzing. Intellectually, most of us still live in a couples' society and couples are more acceptable than singles in many settings. So we're desperate to remain paired. But as relationships get ritualised we gradually lose the habit of taking chances and embracing change. Some wives still choose to make their husbands their career; husbands collude.' One Tory spin doctor, for example, can't bear to socialise unless his wife is present to monitor the introductions and police the small talk – lots of men use women like this as a form of social shield or phantom limb, but even men get tired of the implicit burden of responsibility. Most will ultimately disentangle themselves from women who expect too much dominance.

5 There's the obvious point that if you stop using your right arm it will weaken and wither. The same is true of the capacity to make decisions, to see yourself as a source of authority, to develop a personality in line with your years. It so happens that one of our female neighbours has just been made a judge – now that's what I call getting a message back from society that you've grown up. I don't think she would have achieved this position while acting as a Stepford wife at home. A judge is not a person who asks her husband whether she can please have some money to go shopping. Nor someone who gets romantically taken for granted.

6   In recent times, society has forced its younger members to recognise that a decent standard of living requires two incomes. Likewise, two parents are needed to look after a baby and therefore two adults need to be interchangeable in the money-earning and baby-minding stakes. That siren call 'The pasta is burning, darling!' from an uninvolved male walking past the cooker is definitely Non-U in a modern household. Likewise, women realise that it's growing unacceptable to say 'I never mend punctures' or 'I don't look under car bonnets' or assume that there's always going to be some man to change the light bulbs and replace fuses. The modern youth ideal is *interdependence* and it's a model we could all copy. Emotionally, we sometimes need to be a parent to our partner in order to ensure that they can return the favour when required. But an adult relationship is a deal. Break the deal and the relationship is off. Men are increasingly attracted to women who can handle an electric drill, set up a Web page, talk ecology and bake cookies.

7   No sensible adult should curb their freedom of movement on the grounds that 'he doesn't like me to go out by myself'. Forging intimacy and closeness with other people is a sensible, necessary investment in your personal security, not a covert recipe for adultery. The social reality is that nearly half of all cohabiting relationships break up within four years, one third of all new marriages end in divorce within five years and all human life stops in death eventually. The chance of you and your partner dying at the same time is remote and the chance of you and your partner becoming immortal is zero. Men die on average nine years before women. Yet the 'too-tight' couple still act as if they planned to live forever. Janet and Roger would say 'We will always have each other, won't we?' to which the answer is 'No, you won't!'. Failing to invest in a few close personal friendships is as foolish as never taking out insurance. Boredom thrives on fear. If you retain an independent life in parallel with the intimate partnership the partnership will benefit. You'll have something to talk about!

8 But nor does this mean that you cannot prefer your loved one's company on those special occasions. The relationship between Aubrey and Sarah, for instance, might be called 'close' but not 'fused'. Married for over 28 years they still send doting e-mails, suggestive phone calls and pack themselves off to a country pub in Ireland at least four or five times a year 'to be alone'. Yet, they enjoy a legendary social life with huge parties and lots of time for friends.

9 Research suggests that too-tight partnerships are generally formed by people who've had broken attachments in childhood. Under-parented children, it appears, turn into over-dependent husbands and wives. And over-parented children become even more over-dependent husbands and wives like Janet and Roger. You're lucky if

IS YOURS AN OVER-DEPENDENT RELATIONSHIP?

The presence of four or more of the following should act as a warning:

- extreme jealousy
- failure to make a move without consulting the other
- constant search for approval
- self-victimisation
- routine use of childlike body-language ('Dianism')
- social phobia and social avoidance
- pretended incompetence ('I can't cook'; 'I don't change lightbulbs')

IF IT IS, WHAT CAN YOU DO ABOUT IT?

- cultivate friends of your own
- develop interests in sport or dancing
- improve your educational skills
- take public-speaking courses
- travel in groups
- learn practical DIY
- try personal therapy.

you fall into the arms of someone as childlike as you but the more common outcome is to attract a dominant bully. So you'd probably be better off getting yourself therapy than a wedding ring. The childhood symptoms – desperate jealousy, terrible possessiveness or rock bottom self-esteem – turn up like bad pennies in later partnerships. One ailing wife even uttered the immortal lines: 'Thank God it's me that's dying and not him because I could *never* have survived alone'. The irony, of course, is that *he* survived with ease finding a replacement for her immediately.

10 The 'fusion' model of marriage is often smugly held to be ideal but can lead to a dependency nightmare for either of the parties. When working as an agony aunt, Anne Hooper recalls getting a letter from a woman of 52 who was going out of her mind with frustration. Her husband had always relied on her for everything but then her aged mum came to live with her too. 'It finally got to the stage that when this woman went to the lavatory one day not only her mother sat outside the door to talk to her but so did her husband and then the dog and cat turned up as well'. Rivka Pomson claims that it's more of an issue for women than men: 'Even though it's decades since wives were regarded as appendages of husbands or fathers with no property or voting rights, we are still consumed by this terrible fear of rejection. It's the "I'll do anything as long as you love me" syndrome. If you're going to have a decent relationship with a man you'll often want to do different things from him and sometimes your timing will be terrible. But resolving these conflicts is at the heart of a relationship. What's the point of living with a human doormat? If you're joined at the hip, I say get a hip replacement'.

THE MAN'S VIEW ON SEX AND PARTNERSHIP

In a nutshell, men would like you to keep sex a little bit separate from the routines of family life. It's a perverse paradox, but they find it depressing that women still tend to link sex with babies, sometimes losing interest in lovemaking because the children have been born. Of course, you must 'stay true to yourself' and children's needs have priority but from a strictly male viewpoint it helps to do any or all of the following:

- As soon as the kids are old enough, be prepared to have them looked after occasionally by your or his mum or a sitter.
- Think of going to a hotel or motel just to make love – in his mind this makes a necessary context for sex separate from the responsibilities of family life.
- Explore games and fantasies, clothes and toys, erotic media and stories.
- Talk sex on the phone if it appeals to you both.
- Make love in new places.
- Remember what you did in courtship – enjoy oral sex as well as intercourse, petting as much as penetrating.
- Touch him and get him aroused when it's slightly socially embarrassing.
- Make the bedroom itself comfortable for lovemaking.
- Avoid bringing the children into your bed at night.

IS THERE SEX AFTER MARRIAGE?

Before the wedding, there's lots of lovemaking. 'First sex at marriage is now practically unknown' says the mammoth 1994 survey into Britain's sexual habits conducted by the Welcome Foundation. But the *Sunday Times* has reported that after marriage 'thousands of couples have spurned sex in favour of celibacy'. A previously unpublished *Survey of Sexual Attitudes and Lifestyles* claims that 'up to one in 30 of all couples are opting for celibacy in their relationships because they have neither the time nor the inclination … '

If more than three per cent of us never make love, you can be sure an even bigger percentage don't get much. One lady of a certain age said in a recent episode of the TV detective *Morse*: 'It happens so rarely, Chief Inspector, one *never* forgets the time or place … '

Frequency of sex in the early days depends on temperament and libido but most couples appear to start out with thrice-weekly lovemaking, declining to once a week or fortnight by Year 2. A minority begin by making love up to five times daily and even after several years this only dwindles to about three times a week.

However, it's all too easy for your love-life to succumb to the pressures of habit, commitment and – ultimately – to parenthood. Men probably have more difficulty here because they are less directed to children and sometimes feel less rewarded by children. Obviously, you won't relish daily intercourse throughout a pregnancy (especially in the first and last trimesters and soon after giving birth). But a wise woman makes hay in her middle months while offering comfort and relief at other times.

Equally, don't be surprised if your partner wants *more* sex when there's *more* conflict. For a man, emotional healing takes place as a result of having sex whereas, for a woman, the emotional healing often needs to come first. Some men cannot be touched – physically or emotionally – until they make love. One client said to us: 'When she rejected my lovemaking, she rejected me. I left with a capital 'F' for 'Fail' stamped on my forehead'.

As we have said, most surveys of sexual frequency conclude that committed couples in their late 30s and early 40s rarely make love more than twice a week. This has been a familiar result ever since the post-war Kinsey report. However, only God knows how often people really make love. Many researchers are beginning to think some of the research data is false – with couples exaggerating their frequency rates for fear of being thought unattractive or dull. In effect, women seem to under-report how often they have sex outside marriage and over-report the rates within. It was notable that the *Sunday Times* couldn't get 'Mrs Susan Richards' to use her real name and presumably she wants her friends and family to assume she has a love life when she doesn't.

RELATIONSHIP PATTERNS

So, leaving statistics to their dismal fate, what about relationship patterns? Is there a frequency cycle for sex in a marriage or cohabiting partnership? Answer – yes, (though always leave room for the odd exception). First of all, frequency declines with age – up to two thirds of all men are impotent by the age of 70, a trend that begins at 50. As we have noted, there's a well-documented 'honeymoon phase' in courtship, when sex tends to be an urgent preoccupation. Ethologist Desmond Morris describes this as a bonding ritual using sex for discovery, reassurance and mutual possession. Alas, the sooner it works, the less we need to make love. There is also a psychological law of diminishing returns concerning the 'novelty factor'. This means that the more often you receive a stimulus the less strongly you respond to it. Once we grow familiar with each other's charms we may be less motivated to enjoy them. Then there is a limit to the physical things you can do in bed – we believe it was 47 at the last count.

Here's where patterns become more confusing. There are some souls (a handful, we suspect) for whom the honeymoon phase lasts for life. For most of us, it endures for between nine months and a year. Be warned – you must time this from the moment you first go to bed together, not from your wedding day. Most people are by definition Mr and Mrs Average in the middle – a few people are sexpots or celibate at either end of the chart. And here's where the trouble begins.

When does infrequent sex become not enough sex? When does hardly any sex become no sex? Again, the answer has to be qualified because there are as many types of marriage as there are people. There are also many types of sex from mental to manual. But for 90 per cent of people under 50, complete celibacy *doesn't seem to work*. When sex declines to less than once a month – regardless of cause – most relationships appear to be at risk. Absence of sex is a litmus test; when things turn acid you know it.

NO SEX AT ALL

But how can you tell when a sex-free period has become a sex drought? Well, you must eliminate the common reasonable factors. Are you having a baby? The first three months of pregnancy and sometimes the later months usually put the blocks on. So does post-natal and any other kind of depression. The research shows that children are the perfect combined contraceptive and passion-killer. Is there any illness, emotional disturbance, job insecurity, a loss of sympathy and mutual respect in the family to explain the coolness? If there is, do not expect sex to make things better. It's more common for people to avoid intimacy altogether than find the confidence to 'make it better in bed'. If sex is still not happening, has the relationship fundamentally changed without you realising; is someone having an affair? Is there a deeper game being played – perhaps you are being punished for his mother's or his ex-wife's faults? Have you grown too busy to make time and space for love? We find the crazy world of modern work is behind much of the so-called celibacy boom. In sex therapy, it's not finding the clitoris that's the problem but finding the time to use it.

One couple we counselled never laid a finger on each other yet spent the final two years of their marriage pretending to each other that there wasn't a problem. They continued to sleep in the marital bed, were affectionate last thing at night and early in the morning but gradually learned to make themselves sexually unavailable. She would play a lot of sport and he would get lost on the Internet (yes, looking at erotic pictures). She even came off the Pill in order to start a family but neither of them confronted the basic rules of baby-making. Month after month passed and they both managed to ask for sex when they knew the other person couldn't do it – for reasons of time or tiredness. A painful awakening led to major rows and separation. This wasn't a case of madness – just two people colluding when all passion was spent. Some people fake orgasms; they faked intercourse and we're sure if you'd asked them at the height of this *folie à deux* how often they made love they would have said 'regularly'.

Whatever the case, remember that withholding or withdrawing from sex is a form of communication in itself. Actions speak louder than words. When Mark was 25, he wanted to end things with his girlfriend but couldn't tell her because she had her Oxford finals in three months' time. So he stopped making love to her. Fortunately, she dumped him first, six weeks later – but he honestly didn't how else to act. When people stop making love – unless they've got a valid explanation (which makes sense to *you*) they are trying to tell you that intimacy feels more dangerous than desirable. It is possible to live without – to be celibate like the three per cent in the surveys – but it puts enormous pressure on other forms of contact. If you want to put a figure on it – we'd say that you need to tell someone they're fabulous, and you love them to pieces, about *thirty times a week* to compensate for the absence of sex.

Celibacy also carries the risk of self-delusion. Author Liz Hodgkinson once wrote a book in praise of celibacy in marriage. It wasn't too long afterwards that she got a divorce. If our inner need for attention and respect isn't satisfied, remember that we're programmed like missiles to seek an appointment with destiny – perhaps with Wilf from accounts, or Madge from catering.

On the other hand, there is nothing so simple as fulfilling sex provided you can just make the time and space for your partner. We've known several couples who re-discovered their libidos once the children left home (or were old enough to stay out really late). And we shall never forget Bill and Elaine who wrote to ask if there was an age limit for having real orgasms? She was 72, he was 74. Both had been previously married to partners who had died after long and successful unions. Bill then succumbed to impotence. Within weeks, Bill had been 'brought back from the dead' by Elaine who is now having climaxes of such intensity and duration she wanted to ask if they were physically safe. Moral – sometimes there's so much sex after marriage it can blow your mind but you may have to wait for your pension.

MIS-MATCHED LIBIDO

But how do you tackle it when your two ideas of sex clash or you experience different levels of desire?

frequency:

As we've suggested, relationships usually begin with a bang and then go quiet. You move from loads of sex to a lot less. Men usually claim to be highly-sexed but that should be taken with a pinch of salt. In the honeymoon phase of a new relationship they are generally all over you and eager to prove themselves. Michael, for example, boasted that when they got married he and wife Angela made love 'every day for a year'. But his current sexual position is different. Mike admits he and Angela make love only twice a month 'when circumstances permit'. This is all very irritating for Angela. She feels helpless and loses her confidence.

sex drive:

For biological reasons, nearly all women over the age of consent are capable of having more sex than most male adults. God gave women multiple climaxes while men suffer the 'refractory period'. But these differences tend to obscure people's reasons for wanting or refusing sex. Is he physically spent or not in the mood because you've upset him? Nor are drive and desire the same thing. A woman may never want to make love to her husband but be desperate to leap on a lover, and her lover may feel the same way about his spouse.

Scientists like Britain's first Professor of Sexual Medicine Dr Alan J. Riley say that there are different levels of expectation concerning drive – and a natural distribution curve to go with it. So it's perfectly normal for a few people to want sex all the time and a few people to want sex never. The rest of us come naturally in-between. (This being so, it makes sense to select a partner from a similar point on the curve. A few pertinent questions could be asked early in the relationship).

But, even in the best regulated houses, occasionally your libido and his libido will conflict. Sometimes this is a friendly clash. Life's been hectic. You're feeling neglected. But sometimes it's like the collision of a liner with an iceberg. What you expect from sex and what he expects have nothing in common besides the wrong sort of friction. At the back of your mind are the worst scenarios. Is he seriously depressed? Does he love me any more? Is there A. N. Other?

Pioneering sexologist Dr Robert Chartham said: 'It's impossible to sustain sexual interest by doing the same things in bed in the same way with the same person for the rest of your days. Even changing the colour of the sheets is a help.' Routine sex tends to establish a pattern you could follow in your sleep and sometimes do. Men are especially at fault for becoming what he used to call 'sex lazy'. This is apt to happen after they've persuaded a woman to fall in love and yield to them. Then they stop bothering to impress. Foreplay becomes perfunctory. The woman no longer looks forward to sex. It's not rewarding. The man, sensing rebuff, grows insensitive and selfish and we arrive at that non-erotic one-liner: 'What's an orgasm, Mum?' 'No idea – ask your father'.

But men, too, will get terminally bored so long as we go on pretending sex is really just a male drive. Surely one of the most depressing lines in the English language is 'I never refused him sex' because, by admission, it means that you never demanded any either. Nor have you put your mind to flattery, inventiveness and lust. What is libido if not an expression of something for which there are many words (some more or less acceptable) including horny, randy, twitchy, nervous, desirous, desperate, on the edge and positively gagging for it? Or moody, tempestuous, romantic, thrilling, entrancing, empowering and positively desperate for a night with Mr D'Arcy? The late broadcaster Jill Dando defined one of her love affairs as 'very DH Lawrence'.

sexual styles:

The third element in mis-matched libido is whether your personally preferred style of lovemaking fits with his. In sex therapy, we've come across clients who could only have orgasms while standing, or listening to country music, or after three glasses of wine and an endless kiss. We've also met those who can only be excited if they are first dominated. We personally don't think it matters if you make love trussed like poultry, so long as you and your partner both get something out of it.

Small sexual cues tend to control big sexual responses – the feel of skin on skin, the way a person smiles, how they walk. Get it wrong, the ship will sink. And we haven't even mentioned whether the potential partner kisses like a god or shares your sexual fantasies. On a recent TV programme, a white middle-class woman was pictured meeting a paid 'escort' with whom she might or might not 'take things further' later that night. Afterwards, she confessed: 'I was immediately put off by his body language and suggestive small talk. I didn't like the way he related to women – for example, he called them "ladies". I couldn't begin to fancy him. He was the wrong type and the wrong class for me.' If this man could have spoken differently suggestive of a different social background she might happily have said 'Yes'.

PUTTING THINGS RIGHT
This will involve up to five basic re-assessments.

your sexual contract:
We all have one. The contract is either conscious or assumed. Built in is the idea of frequency. We generally know when there hasn't been enough contact lately. And from time to time, you need to sit down with your partner and carry out an audit. You look at your excuses. See how busy life is. Weigh up your priorities. If you really are investing more time in watching soap operas or being Treasurer of the local Golf Club than in having sexual intercourse, ask yourself 'Is this for the best?' Television hath charms and distracts but it will never love you back. Perhaps ask yourself or your partner why the sex has stopped.

make a date for sex:
Or even dates. But don't get alarmed – you never have to have an orgasm if you don't want to. All that's required is that you create time and space for intimacy and the chance for your partner to feel sexual pleasure while sharing your company and caresses. It's private time

without interruptions, with few clothes and lots of candles, warmth, music and skin-on-skin. Every relationship needs routine episodes like these or you've probably lost your direction anyway. If your partner is growing anxious about the future and seeks extra sex as a remedy, here is your chance to steady and regulate the problem.

bring in a third party:

Imagine there's a therapist in your life (a nice one, naturally) who can be that 'third voice' during difficult or contentious moments. When you next fight about sex, this imaginary person can be saying simple things like 'Is this conversation going round in circles?', 'Can you two call a time out now for at least two silent minutes?', 'Would you both stop talking and have a peaceful hug?', 'Could you also see this from your partner's point of view?', and if things are getting totally fraught 'Can you possibly agree to disagree?' Simply by looking at your problems through different spectacles you acquire 'behavioural flexibility'.

take things in turns:

Tonight, he's in charge and perhaps the menu will read 'Chinese meal and video'. Tomorrow, you're in charge and the menu reads 'Baked potatoes and mega-bonk'.

change the environment:

If not much is changing in your love life and the emotional positions seem to be getting more embattled, try changing the environment altogether by going away for sex. Most of us can recapture the spirit of honeymoon in locations where the chores are managed by others and workaday stresses are left behind. If nothing else, you get the freedom to address your differences without interruption. At worst, you will find yourself in bed with a familiar 'stranger'. At best, you'll get complaints from the neighbouring guests.

THE CHRONIC INSECURITY AT
THE HEART OF MALE SEXUALITY

If none of these approaches works quickly, then you may have to consider the deeper psychological implications of masculine sexual anxiety. How many men do you think suffer clinically from sex problems?

Jack says: 'I love my
girlfriend and we have
great sex but there's
always tension. Sometimes
she gets carried away and
begs me to come during
foreplay or when we've
just started intercourse.
Then she goes "Oh Gosh"
because she knows I
won't be able to manage
another erection for a
couple of hours and she's
hardly got started and
was really eager for more.
I do the best I can
manually – manfully, in
the circumstances – but
we both realise it's my
second best.'

The answer is about 90 per cent fewer than those who've ever joked about taking Viagra. James, a 42-year-old investment broker with no history of sexual difficulties and a good marriage explains why he keeps a few of the blue diamond-shaped capsules in his medicine chest: 'As a bloke it's always good to know you've got backup...'

This persistent rumble of insecurity at the heart of male sexuality begins with the biological basics. In love, a man must stand up and be counted – or be counted out. 'When I have sex with my wife,' says Jack, a 33-year-old forestry worker, 'there's always that nagging uncertainty that desire will fail – and no way on the planet can I conceal my lack of interest.'

It's an ancient theme, of course, but if God really wanted to have a little male joke when deciding how the two sexes should mate – He succeeded. Male sexuality is principally rooted in the old, dinosaur part of the brain rather than the modern computer section. There's a lumbering train of reflexes shunting blood from other parts of the body into the empty spaces of the penis by hormonal control. The erection system relies on old-style hydraulics, not muscles. In other words, a man can always raise his hand in the air to caress his partner but must wait for the right time, place, and circumstances, and enough fantasy and friction, before his penis will do the same. At root, male sexual response is essentially passive …

Anxiety is to men what rain is to Wimbledon. All play gets suspended. Till lately, doctors didn't know how 'worry' could cause loss of virility. Now they've found the culprit in old-fashioned adrenaline. As a man grows anxious during sex, a kick of adrenaline causes his penile valves to lock in the 'open' position. It's just like a canal lock that won't close. What's more, local blood pressure cannot rise again until the anxious feeling and its aftermath have both been allowed to pass. So the more a man worries about being able to perform the more certain it is that he can't.

MALE BELIEFS ABOUT MANHOOD

Of course, there's a reason why early dinosaurs *wanted* to confine their sexual operations to moments of complete safety. Terrible things can happen when your back is turned, even to Monstrous Rex. But this battle in men between their basic brain stems and computer forebrains causes endless complications. Computers tend to outwit their own programmers. As long as men can use their frontal lobes to solve problems they can also use them to create them. Some male beliefs about manhood surprise even us.

For instance, there's Alan, a married man of 27: 'My wife and I went through a really rocky patch. Most of it was my fault but we drifted apart for a few weeks and during that time she had a one-night stand. I couldn't cope with this. I began to imagine I'd become gay. Here was a lovely sexy girl, willing to dress up in any way I wanted and I couldn't respond. It had to mean I preferred guys.'

Or take, Martin, a 31-year-old marketing executive: 'Ever since puberty I've been worried about the size of my manhood. I now realise I'm probably about average but the problem is that, after years of anxiety over size and more important over performance, I suffer from impotency problems. I've learnt to be sensitive to women's needs and manage to bring my partners to orgasm with foreplay and I quite enjoy this build-up of tension but I just can't sustain an erection for very long and this brings me down.'

Women, of course, are often on the non-receiving end. Jess, a solicitor, says: 'I was more than a little dismayed when he couldn't manage the tiniest bulge of interest.' And Rachel, a property manager, adds: 'The first night he said "I guess I'm over-excited." On the second night he said: "Oh dear, not again!" On the third night he said: "I don't understand, this has never happened to me before." On the fourth night he said: "It's definitely not you – it's that me *not* getting an erection has now become too important." I felt I wasn't womanly enough. Eventually it emerged that he was having a specific problem at work. When that was settled (his boss got transferred) the impotence more or less cured itself but it was too late for me.'

IT'S HARDER FOR BOYS

Psychoanalysis suggests that finding an effective sexual identity *is* harder for boys. Whereas girls can cheerfully grow up into a version of their mums, boys who do this turn into casualties. Society expects junior men to 'make the journey to the other side', away from mum's femininity towards father's darker maleness. This is difficult if father is parked up at the pub or being prosecuted by the Child Support Agency. *It's a hard task, anyway.* Even in happy families, boys must leave the warm safety of the maternal bosom and opt for that lonely swim into the outside world. Some men take their protests to an extreme.

Bernard, a 28-year-old taxi driver – who on his days off likes to be known as Bernadette, in a fetching Versace number – is angry that men who cross-dress are ridiculed whereas the same sartorial rules never apply to women. He means that if Margaret Thatcher had chosen to wear trousers in Parliament no one would care whereas Prime Minister Blair in a frock would lose his job. New Labour, Same Old Suits. For men under pressure there's nowhere to hide, not even within the concealing whirls of a generous skirt!

From a woman's perspective, the task is to see through men's misleading PR. The spin is hardly sophisticated. Men say that they can face anything. They mean that they wished they dared. They say they're never worried by failure. They mean the precise opposite. They pretend they've had loads of sexual experience. They mean they haven't read a single book on female anatomy. Ask for directions? 'Real men don't do that.' In one television survey, 67 per cent of men couldn't identify the location of the clitoris on a map of the female body. The truth is that male claims are compensations – generally, they are sexually shy, introverted and fundamentally relieved that they've invented Viagra. So, if your man is showing signs of flagging sexual self-confidence, boost him with encouragement, information and loving understanding. Beneath male boasting and bluster is fear. Beneath the fear is depression. And beneath that, in the middle of the male psyche, is an awareness of the terror of rejection – the sexual consequences of which we examine in Chapter Four.

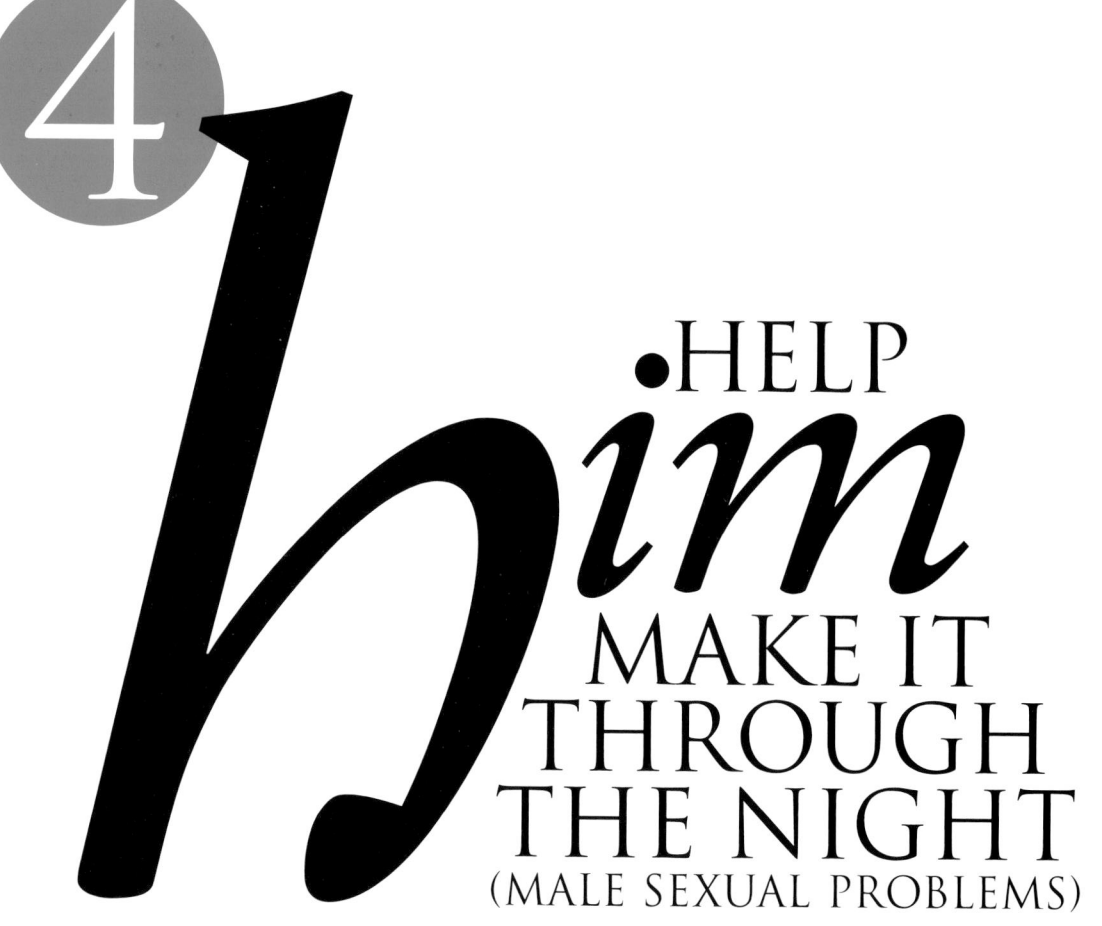

4

HELP him MAKE IT THROUGH THE NIGHT
(MALE SEXUAL PROBLEMS)

Sometimes a man cannot possibly do what a man has to do. But a good woman can help him overcome the common imperfections which flesh is heir to. At some stage in his life your dismayed lover may find that he's got a sex problem. This is highly likely because from time to time it is normal for a man to fail to get an erection. Younger men regularly climax too quickly. On rare occasions and especially when first launching into a love life, some guys find it very hard to climax at all. So please expect to become a soothing friend and sex therapist on the predictable occasions when this occurs.

COPING WITH IMPOTENCE

The poet John Betjeman suffered ('My sex is no longer rampant'). Sir Anthony Buck apparently suffered ('It took two years for the marriage to be consummated to wife Bienvenida'). Even James Bond has suffered ('For an hour in that room alone with Le Chiffre the certainty of impotence had been beaten into him and a scar had been left that could only be healed by experience'). A pity they didn't live to see the current trend of impotence research and development.

We all know about Viagra (that compound word which is a blend of 'vigour' and the Niagara Falls). It is now possible to deliver a user-friendly chemical to overcome the difficulties of impotence in up to 70 per cent of cases. Medically-speaking, this is a huge number – very few pills in any field of doctoring can make a claim approaching this figure. But the compound also produces some unwanted side effects: it is not usable by patients with heart conditions and it is by no means an aphrodisiac. You have to wait up to an hour for the penis to respond and you still need to conduct foreplay. One New York couple took the pill, waited for action then fell asleep in frustration – having forgotten to lay hands on each other! As a result of these and similar difficulties, Viagra is no longer regarded as the golden panacea. Uptake in the UK has been far less than expected and the surge of consumption in the USA is dropping off.

Even so, it *should* be an exciting time for erections. There is an entire range of new products available or in the pipeline to help most men. However, one recent survey of 432 patients and 194 partners published on behalf of the UK Impotence Association was significantly deflating. The Chairman of the Association, Dr Alan J. Riley, says that up to five million British men suffer from some form of 'erectile dysfunction' *yet only 10% receive any form of treatment.* Of those seeking help, one in four neglects to visit their doctor – preferring to trust to commercial alternatives such as sprays, herbs and 'energy rings'. Of those who do visit the surgery, 23% get no treatment whatsoever. Of those who do visit the doctor and get treatment, a massive 58% come away dissatisfied:

- 62% of sufferers overall reported lowered self-esteem and some feelings of depression.
- 15% had trouble making new relationships.
- 14% said impotence had damaged their long-term partnerships.
- 10% thought it had even spoiled their relationship with the doctor.
- 25% of the respondents said that impotence reduced their overall quality of life by up to 80%.

Allan Bennet, in his 50s, is typical of those who express frustration with the system: 'I have had sexual difficulties for more than two years. Reluctantly, I went to see my GP having finally plucked up the courage. He asked me what I expected at my age and did it really matter any more? I'd got my family, hadn't I? And with a magisterial wave he dismissed my concerns. I was so flabbergasted I remained speechless. The doctor in question, I might add, is a Roman Catholic. It was only when I got home that my brain jogged back into gear. I sent him the following note:

> *Dear Doctor,*
>
> *I know that you have indicated that the virility problem is not of fundamental importance to the continuation of my marriage but I can assure you that it most definitely is vital to the continued existence of my peace of mind as a man. I thought you should be informed I shall be seeing a sexual consultant in London …*

When you consider that good sex adds years to the life of middle-aged men like Allan, cutting the risk of premature death by as much as 36% per 100 orgasms, this does amount to a legitimate health concern. Yet time and again for reasons of embarrassment or lack of empathy, GPs seem reluctant to prescribe.

HEALTH AND IMPOTENCE

Up to a third of men over 45 experience some symptoms of impotence and up to two thirds of those aged 75. Longer life-span usually means more heart and hypertension problems. These may cause impotence directly, or as a result of taking medication. The same is true of depression – a common enough feature of mid-life. Both the illness and remedies such as Prozac can reduce libido and affect sexual performance. New drugs to counteract baldness such as Propecia also carry some impotence risk.

SMOKES AND BOOZE

Nor do old drugs like alcohol and nicotine help. Men who consume more than 40 units of booze a week are likely to deliver little or no sexual thrill. It's been shown that smoking two high-tar cigarettes, one after the other, reduces blood-flow in the penis by about a third. And the perennial campaign to promote Cannabis has to answer concerns that up to 20 per cent of long-term cannabis-users may become impotent.

Even if you're trying to lead a drug-free, well-exercised lifestyle, there's little prospect of escape. The latest significant cause of impotence among younger men turns out to be 'bicycle-riding', at least according to Dr Irwin Goldstein of Dallas, Texas (his website: http://www.nd.edu/~ktrembat/www-bike/BCY/men.bikes.html), who sees six such patients per week. He claims that that hard saddles on sports' bikes are responsible for reducing penile blood flow by up to 66% and even the softer versions reduce blood supply to the region by a third.

IMPOTENCE REMEDIES

So it's just as well we live in a period replete with remedies. We've mentioned Viagra. But injectable prostaglandins like Caverject are a special boon for diabetes and stroke patients. Men cross their legs when you mention injections but the sensation is said to be no more than a 'small prick', according to Dr Geoff Hackett of Keele University who ran tests for five years. To those critics who say doctors are yet again 'interfering with nature' he replied: 'Spontaneous intercourse isn't very common in most 20-year-old marriages. My studies show that 39 per cent of patients with diabetes are permanently impotent. Over 50 per cent of stroke patients are impotent. And most of those with spinal damage who can't walk and have sometimes little else to live for are impotent. Not only will many of these sufferers be able to resume sexual activity, the quality of their erections is likely to exceed anything they've experienced since boyhood.' Another version of this compound (called MUSE) is available in pellet form for needle-phobes.

In addition to these treatments, there is a vast array of hard or semi-hard penile rods and implants some with external bulb-inflators, which may be fitted by a plastic surgeon, in addition to hand-applied pumps, splints and bands. But in all this discussion of prosthetics and sexual chemistry where is the human touch?

Already we have a consumer-friendly alpha-1 blocker impotence remedy (called *Erecnos*) which, unlike Caverject and MUSE, does *not* induce erection in the absence of sexual stimulation. But popping a pill is never going to be the complete answer. Men, after all, are only half the equation. We already know that more than one third of the partners of impotent men have sexual problems of their own, so marital and sexual counselling is more important, not less, in this age of wonder drugs.

PREMATURE EJACULATION

Premature ejaculation is another widespread, quite easily treated sexual difficulty which can ruin anyone's evening. Nothing is biologically wrong with most men who come 'too quickly'. This can be maddening for dissatisfied partners and sufferers seeking a quick fix. But the purpose of sex is pregnancy and for that seconds will do. When early man mounted early woman he didn't hang around. He jumped then humped. The result was like Angie Dickinson's description of her seduction by President Kennedy: 'The most memorable fifteen seconds of my life'.

The Male Health Center of Dallas, Texas, claims that premature ejaculation (PE) is a problem affecting 25 per cent of all men 'if it is defined as ejaculation within five minutes'. But why should we do that? You could equally say PE is a *relationship* problem as the Rev E. Lyttelton did writing to sex therapist Marie Stopes in 1920:

'You emphasise ... that gratification should be shared by the female ... but the difficulty must often be that the discharges do not coincide in time. If that of the woman is late, it is difficult to see what ought to be done, as to prolong intercourse would be for the man a serious strain ...' Quite so.

Far from there being anything wrong with those who rush, men could ask why do females need so long to get started? If a woman in a good relationship requires one hour of intercourse to reach orgasm, should the man be called 'premature' because he comes after 45 minutes? You might say 'Yes'. The man might say 'You must be bloody joking!'

Most men want to please their lovers. They realise that 'nice guys finish last', as Leo Durocher once said of the New York Giants. They'll do all they can to deliver the goods ... delightfully late. But don't start off by making your man feel guilty just because God screwed up the server system.

HAS YOUR MAN EVER SUFFERED FROM PE?

Of course he has. Men begin their love lives as premature ejaculators and suffer further bouts with new girlfriends into their 20s. As we've said, sex hormone levels rise by a massive per cent during adolescence. Then men discover what happens between their legs. They tend to play with any new toy a lot. In this particular case, they are equally anxious not to be observed while doing so. It means the resulting sexual style of most young men is a blur of nerves and speed.

Masturbation is destiny. Compared to a vagina, the human fist can move faster than a Japanese bullet train. Men tend to condition themselves to sprints then grow disturbed during intercourse when they discover they lack control. Conditioning goes deeper if your man discovered sex in the cinema and experimented in the back seats of cars with a constant fear of interruption. As for those who pay to lose their virginity – for prostitutes, time is always money.

SO WHEN DOES PE BECOME A PROBLEM?

Only when you can't be satisfied! In its most severe form, a PE male climaxes *before* any direct stimulation of the penis has occurred. Just thinking about a sexually stimulating situation triggers ejaculation. This is rare. It is much more common for ejaculation to take place either *during* or a few seconds *after* penetration of the vagina. Some women suffer the same 'hair trigger' trouble as men. Faye Dunaway's character in the movie *Network* wanted to get showered and dressed before Peter Finch, her partner, had managed to break sweat. Other women climax from nipple caresses alone. Presumably with such a girlfriend, a premature ejaculator could have an *entirely compatible* relationship?

HOW COMMON IS PE?

PE is still the most common sexual problem affecting men, according to the UK Impotence Association. Research suggests that one man in ten experiences severe or occasional impotence but as many as four men in ten are troubled by PE on more than an occasional basis. To a great extent, the young are more affected than the old because PE is related to the novelty of the sexual experience (more new partners, environments) rather than to age. But the good news is that PE remains the easiest sexual problem to cure.

WHAT HAPPENS DURING NORMAL EJACULATION?

You'd think that after all this time the experts would be able to tell us. But they say the human sexual system is really difficult to map. However, ejaculation appears to be a three-stage process. After arousal, a small bead of fluid may appear at the penile tip. This may come from Cowper's gland or be shed through the lining of the urethra. It may or may not contain a few sperm leaking from the testes (accounting for a few unplanned pregnancies). Second, liquid from the prostate gland plus sperm from the coiled tubes of the testicles is moved by automatic transmission into a sort of holding tank or storage siding and the internal bladder sphincter closes off. So far, a man feels cocky but not really out of control.

The Big Fun Stage Three begins when the external bladder sphincter flips open allowing the fluid to drain into the urethral bulb. Ejaculation proper involves passing the 'point of no return' or 'moment of ejaculatory inevitability'. Your man is going to come and nothing in the world – not even a mad gunman saying he'll shoot him if he does – can stop it. A delicious delay of three seconds is followed by the discharge of all the fluid in powerful contractions of the Kegel muscles at 0.8 second intervals propelling the ejaculate for a distance of up to 60 cms (so some of the writing on toilet walls is true).

WHAT HAPPENS DURING PE?

In a nutshell, premature ejaculators cannot distinguish between two distinct sets of feelings – the moment before orgasm (when ejaculation can still be prevented) and the actual 'point of no return' (when it can't). The key process is the opening of the external bladder sphincter, which needs to be consciously monitored. Just as all men learn to close this sphincter at age two and a half to avoid wetting the bed, so now they need to learn to delay opening it in the interests of better sex. This is partly a matter of reviewing their own state of arousal, seeing when you need to ease up on the accelerator, and partly about exercising their buttock muscles.

IS ANXIETY THE ROOT OF THE PROBLEM?

The biggest living name in sex research on both sides of the Atlantic, Dr John Bancroft, currently at the Kinsey Institute, Indiana, says 'yes' and

ONE ORGASM OR MANY?

It Is also possible to release the ejaculate *without* pleasurable contractions in a process termed emission which can be triggered by a urological massage. There are also oriental philosophers who claim that ejaculation and orgasm are not the same thing although if the sphincter does not open this is hard to believe.

thinks that how men label their fears affects their biochemistry. Put simply, fear of success causes PE, never fear of failure. If your man expects to over-succeed, he *will* over-succeed whereas if he expects to fail, he'll fail. In the former case, 'positive' anxiety *enhances* sexual response. In the latter case, 'negative' anxiety can even make him lose his erection.

HOW WOULD POSITIVE ANXIETY EXAGGERATE PE?

In the human body, all nervous impulses have to use the same pathways. Growing anxious and getting turned on provoke similar responses – raised temperature, rapid pulse, red face, dry mouth, butterflies in the stomach. Premature ejaculators are by definition more anxious and self-conscious than the rest. So what they fail to realise is how far their anxiety level has already aroused them. The horse is practically galloping before the race has started. Worry is foreplay, so it only takes the excitement of penetration to cause climax.

WHAT DOES WORK?

The first thing to remember, says Dr Mike Perring of Optimal Health of Harley Street, who specialises in sexual problems, is to help him avoid panic. A good self-help book on relaxation and breathing exercises can be worth its weight in gold. The second is to choose simple solutions first. 'If the difficulty persists for a very young man who has an inexperienced partner and he's not a chronic sufferer, it's sometimes a help for him to masturbate before making love. Everyone knows that the second time always takes longer so having got the first time out of the way it gives the opportunity to make seconds a real delight. And a young man can probably come twice fairly quickly. Even nicer, of course, if his partner does the masturbating for him … '

The general wisdom among therapists is that getting your man to distract his mind by thinking of his tax forms or applying an anaesthetic spray to the offending organ is pointless. The therapeutic goal is to make the patient more aware of his sensations, not less. He needs to gain better knowledge about the 'moment of no return' and reduce stimulation till the danger subsides. It's counter-productive to encourage his mind to wander or to drug his penis. He needs more sensory focus, not dope.

WAYS *NOT* TO TREAT PE

Here's a list of things that **don't** work:

- long-term psychoanalysis
- getting drunk
- using two condoms
- him concentrating on something other than sex while having sex
- him biting your cheek
- testosterone injections
- tranquillisers

A THERAPY TALE

There's an old joke about a businessman in bed with his secretary saying: 'Of course I ejaculate prematurely. I'm a very busy man!' One sex-therapy client reminded us of this when he arrived with his wife for help with the problem of PE. Whenever we asked her a question, he would cut in with the answer. It was almost impossible for him to stop taking responsibility for everything going on around him or connected with his marriage and family. When we asked about the rest of his life, it emerged he buzzed around the office like a bluebottle, always broke the speed limit in his car and gobbled his food. When we got him to be silent, he heard that his partner was displeased with more than their sex life. We began to work on their conflicts. He discovered that his wife had wishes of her own, previously unexpressed. He began to hear from her that it takes two to make love in an equal partnership. He learned from us how to stop being a very busy man in bed. Gradually, he got in touch with his own sexual feelings, instead of hearing an order to 'be the dutiful conjugal leader'. Having grasped that it is not an essential part of the male role to run the sexual show, this man also learned that he was not, ultimately, bound to take responsibility for his wife's orgasm; he needed instead to look after his own. Sex, he began to see, is not something men do to women but something men and women share. He says he is a happier man today (who can last as long as he likes during sex); he has resigned as conjugal leader and no longer threatens his penis with death if it falls asleep on duty.

DRUGS AND OTHER TREATMENTS

Professor Alan Riley says: 'Unfortunately, most of the products sold in sex shops or by mail order have not been properly evaluated. Only one product has been approved by the UK Ministry of Health for the treatment of premature ejaculation and that's called Stud 100, an anaesthetic spray. Drugs taken by mouth which delay ejaculation such as paroxetine and sertraline are available and are being found useful in the treatment of premature ejaculation when other approaches fail.' Some anti-depressants tend to reduce libido and potency so the beneficial effect on PE is cancelled out. It's also possible to gain indirect benefit from impotence treatments such as Caverject which prolong erection regardless of ejaculation.

KEGEL THERAPY

Toning the pubococcygeal, or Kegel, muscles is another useful step in reducing the chances of PE, according to many of the Internet gurus. Clearly it's easier to flex a well-honed area of tissue than a flabby no-go zone. To find his Kegels, your man should sit in a chair and try to wiggle his penis without touching it – the muscles he is sitting on are the ones to exercise and they extend to the base of the penis. He can practise anywhere.

WHAT YOU CAN DO TO HELP

It *is* possible for him to break the habits of a lifetime with the aid of a sympathetic partner. There are several sex-therapy approaches you can try at home – including the Start/Stop, the Squeeze Technique or the Beautrais Manoeuvre.

START/STOP

First, the start-stop, which has a 90 per cent success rate. When in bed together, get him to masturbate for a few minutes and then, before he is in danger of climaxing, tell him to stop caressing himself and wait till desire dwindles. Then he should resume for another few minutes. Ask him to repeat three times in all before climaxing. He should do this over several nights. When he feels ready – but only then – very gradually take over. Use your own hands, and eventually a lubricant, and masturbate him in the same way as he has previously done. Warn him to say when he thinks the sensations are in danger of causing climax. Instantly remove your hand and passion again is allowed to subside. Repeat three times before letting him climax, again over several nights.

When – and only when – he can manage this without difficulty, graduate to popping his penis into your vagina in the woman-on-top-position. Just keep it there and stay still. You can hold a conversation if you like. Do this several times without moving, on several occasions. It's called 'enclosure' (as opposed to 'penetration') and allows the man to surrender responsibility for the action. When he can manage this successfully over a sequence of nights, then – and only then – start to move gently on his penis. As soon as he thinks his feelings are beginning to run away with him, you can slip yourself off and prevent ejaculation, perhaps using the Squeeze Technique (next).

THE SQUEEZE TECHNIQUE

This is really an extension of the above because as soon as the woman lifts herself off the man's penis she can apply the world-famous 'Squeeze Technique' – the success rate for which is also about 90 per cent. To apply, you place the thumb under the head ridge of the penis and your first two fingers on top then squeeze hard. It won't really hurt since what you are squeezing is a hydraulic tube. But his passion and possibly his erection will ebb. Then start the process over again, and repeat the squeeze. In about six or eight weeks of re-training, you should find any difficulty is remedied and you can both enjoy more spontaneous sex. Note: these weeks are tough on your sexual endurance so make sure you receive plenty of pleasure from his hands and mouth on demand!

THE BEAUTRAIS MANOEUVRE

Otherwise called the 'swerve', this technique was invented by a New Zealand sex therapist called Pierre Beautrais. He was astute enough to notice that during moments of intense sexual arousal a man's testes, like the undercarriage on an aeroplane, rise up towards his body pulled by the delicate cremaster muscles (the same ones that draw his balls into his belly when he feels intensely cold). His experiments showed that when a PE sufferer (or partner) prevented this elevation manually, orgasm could be successfully delayed. It's simply a matter of a man learning to fly with the wheels down.

DELAYED EJACULATION

This condition can be mild or severe, though most men with the problem would fall into the first of these groups. It is rare to come across individuals who have *never* been able to achieve climax. In these milder forms, delayed ejaculation is apparently quite prevalent though firm data is not available.

Ejaculation, as we've said, contains two phases – emission and expulsion. The first allows the seminal fluid to gather inside the base of the penis (the 'arming phase') and is accompanied by no great sensation of pleasure – more a warning of the growing approach of orgasm. The second (the shooting phase) requires the contraction of the striated and bulbar muscles of the perineum and is responsible for the enormous delights which climax can bring.

Unfortunately, this second phase is under the control of the voluntary nervous system so a man may prevent ejaculation because his conscious and unconscious thoughts interfere with the process.

It is also important to consider the role of excess stress in the onset of this condition. A man who is always anxious or holding his muscles rigid is also exerting too much control over his perineal musculature as well and needs to find appropriate forms of general relief and relaxation.

If there has been a history of diabetes, nerve damage, prostatic disease and urethral scarring, ejaculation difficulties may have an entirely physical cause and these factors would need medical investigation. Some prescription drugs including beta-blockers and some anti-depressants may also interfere with the ejaculation process.

PSYCHOLOGICAL FACTORS

Two categories of men would commonly present with the problem of delayed ejaculation. The first would be sex starters who are paralysed with guilt or other strong emotions. The second would be older men who have grown psychologically mistrustful of release, or who have a need for greater physical stimulation now that age has made lovemaking less spontaneous and orgasm less compliant. A typical question might come from the partner of the man affected:

Q I've been going to bed with my boyfriend for five weeks now and he's never been able to climax with me once. Is it me or is it him?

A Men who cannot come inside a woman may have a combination of technique and attitude problems. For instance, many men learn how to do sex by masturbating. When they bring themselves to orgasm, they may agitate with their hands far more quickly than two people can ever have sex. Hence, when they start making love, the sensations seem under-stimulating.

The answer to this part of the problem is to increase the eroticism of foreplay, make your partner wait until he's practically on the edge of climax before allowing him to insert his penis.

If this doesn't help, and you find he has a history of poor female relationships (mother or lover having let him down), then you will have to coax him more gently. Anxiety is preventing him from triggering his ejaculatory reflex. Tell him there is a remedy that you can jointly try over a period of weeks.

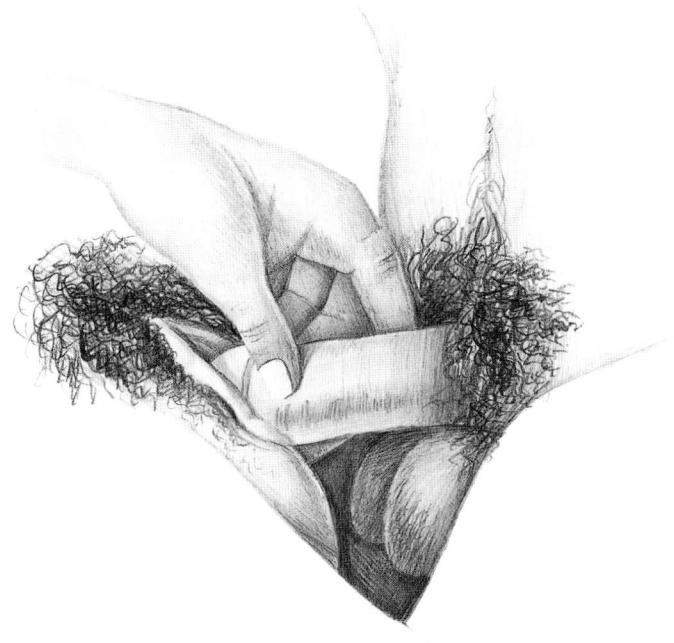

When the time is right, and you are feeling intimate and relaxed, ask him to show you how he masturbates all the way to orgasm. Be light-hearted and make it fun. Next time, ask him to masturbate with a little assistance from you. Next time, see if he can do it just inside your vulva again with assistance from your hand if he enjoys it. At this point, if the process has proved successful, draw his attention to the fact that you are virtually having normal sexual intercourse and that he *has* managed to ejaculate where you both want him to.

On the next occasion, he could insert himself fully and try coming deep inside you – and so on. It may sound a little awkward or even boring but you're wrong. This therapy has great joint potential. And it does work. The important point to remember is that if at any stage he meets with a reverse, you don't fret but simply return to the previous stage and get comfortable with that again. It may also be helpful to ask your partner to describe his fantasies, or to entertain him with your own, or use strong sexual words or images, during the 'treatment' sessions. Some couples prefer to intersperse oral sex with attempts at vaginal sex to heighten the man's arousal.

If the former, does he have
religious-based inhibitions?
Some men were taught that
sex is sinful, or sex before
or outside marriage is
'wrong', or have been
perturbed by female
menstruation or body odour
and it is for these reasons
that they cannot ejaculate.
Gentle coaxing and re-
education may be helpful.
You could challenge some
of the more puritanical
assumptions – for instance,
who created sex if it wasn't
God? Does God really
intend us all to have these
sexual feelings then reject
their self-expression? You
could say the Bible is a
good book but we know for
a fact it was written by
dozens of different authors
over many years telling
hand-me-down stories
many of which display
inner contradictions. Why
do we take literally that
which was written under
such circumstances rather
than glean its 'spirit', which
is that we should care for
one another?

THE TALKING APPROACH

Coupled with these physical therapy approaches, it would also be important to coax your partner into talking about his deep-seated feelings towards sex, women and feminine values. In a nutshell, has he ever been traumatised or 'punished' for engaging in 'forbidden' sexual activities or been abandoned or dumped by important women-figures in the past? If the latter, ask him to describe the specific instance and to share any bottled-up resentments.

Many men with delayed ejaculation have more diffuse concerns. What they really fear is 'letting go', or giving their partner an emotional hold over them since during orgasm it's impossible to 'stay in control'. Again, it would be important under these circumstances, to get the man to practise 'letting go' in many different everyday situations – from being a passenger in a car or plane to playing a blindfold game as part of love-play. If your guy just seems unable to respond to any of this however, drag him off to the doctor and get him a referral to a psychotherapist. Thankfully, such cases are not so common. If the difficulty concerns a wider lack of sexual drive or desire, turn to the next chapter.

5

THE LAND OF lost LIBIDO

You didn't realise libido *could* be lost? Yes, of course it can. Sometimes things gets so bad a man can't even be bothered to wonder whether he'd like any sex – or watch his favourite movie star remove her clothes on screen.

WHAT LIBIDO IS

Most sex therapists find it useful to distinguish between drive and desire: 'Sexual drive is the energy that makes men want to have sexual release; sexual desire is a focused drive: a man desires to have sex with a particular partner. It's perfectly possible to lose desire for a wife, for example, and yet be desperate to go to bed with the next door neighbour. The drive is intact.'

We're all familiar with sexual frustration – the longing that tells you it's really been far, *far* too long. One friend said: 'I'm madly in love with Susie but when she goes away for a week, I stop missing her and start missing *it*'. And some guys have such a high sex-drive they stop at nothing – they'll chat up a melon. But a sudden, complete lack of drive might even indicate a medical condition and should be checked out.

DOES LIBIDO MATTER?

Yes, because sexual satisfaction ultimately depends on feeling that there is a strong drive for sex. A University of Michigan study found that men in their 70s were just as happy with their sex lives as men in their 30s so long as their drive and erections remained intact. This was true regardless of whether they obtained enough sex. It's knowing they want it that counts!

IS GLOBAL MALE SEX-DRIVE FALLING?

The National Opinion Research Center in the USA reports that one out of six younger men experiences a diminishment in his sex-drive that can last several months at a time. But for most people 'this ebb represents a phase'. Not so much fun of course if you're both in the middle of that phase. Here's the bad news. With every decade that passes, the percentage of men feeling a stir of desire more than once a week falls drastically. At 30, libido regularly arouses 80 per cent of men; by age 70, it's fallen to 10 per cent.

WHAT GOES WRONG?

1 It could be falling hormone levels especially of 'free testosterone'. One study of 92 Greek army recruits concluded that those with high free testosterone averaged 11 orgasms per week while the rest managed a paltry 3.9. Dr Malcolm Carruthers, author of *The Andropause*, recommends male hormone replacement therapy as the answer.

2 Professor Alan Riley of Preston University thinks that it is more about state of mind than body. He says we need input to get output: 'Sexual satisfaction depends on sexual desire and desire depends on satisfaction. It's a loop. When a man has great sex he feels reinforced, so he wants more. If sex is a disaster zone, he'll naturally try to avoid intimacy. Sexual satisfaction is a simple equation – "How nearly does what you get out of sex measure up to what you expect"' If his expectation of his performance and partner is sky-high, he'll kill his satisfaction.'

Riley says he personally believes in the Rule of Twos: 'Out of ten acts of intercourse, two may be wonderful, two may be rotten while six may be mediocre'. Having boring sex also stops you wanting sex. If you ate Beluga caviar and roast sucking pig every day you'd soon get sick of it (just like those Scottish serfs who petitioned their lord in 1880 to stop sending them fresh salmon for dinner). Riley thinks sex is the only recreation where people don't plan ahead although we know variety is essential. 'Just lighting candles can give the bedroom a different feel.'

3 Depression also takes over. Losing interest in sex is depressing and depression is a number one passion-killer, says Dr Frank Goodwin of the US National Institute of Mental Health. He believes that depression (including winter S.A.D.) lies behind as many as 30 per cent of cases of lost libido in men. 'Feeling mildly depressed is a normal response to life's curved balls. Clinical depression however is a whole different ball game. Men lose energy because of restless sleep and early morning waking. They gain weight (or lose it) because food tastes like cardboard. Their bodies ache because inner turmoil produces muscular tension. Dating is impossible because they can't take decisions. Alcohol gets abused and that disturbs their sleep patterns all the more.' All glasses in life seem half empty – except for the glass of Scotch in the hand.

4 Conflict in relationships is a definite turn-off. No one wants to get naked with a partner who thinks that the difference between men and batteries is that batteries have a positive terminal. The rows can be about anything – time spent at work, tidiness, money – but the results are the same. The man won't want sex. And you don't want sex. What you really want to do is to feel justified in your anger and be awarded £40 million compensation by a cosmic jury. Then you might feel a bit more like it. So try some self-help measures at solving the problems or even consider formal counselling.

5 Exercise is a sexual puzzle. Those who work out a lot report a fabulous sex life and rock-hard libido. But some overdo it. For every marathon man who lasts all night there are one or two who lose interest. Horizontal jogging is, after all, just jogging and, if your man has already done 10 miles, he may not want to move another 10 inches.

6 Over-stress is a prime libido-killer. The reason, says psychologist Dr Eamon McGann, is that the human system must 'alternate between tension and relaxation if it is to be efficient, if it is to grow and, in fact if it is to survive'. Tension, it seems, is necessary to life – without it there can be no behaviour. A life without stress is actually called death. 'It is not tension that kills human desire,' says McGann, 'it is continual tension without relief. That's why electronic information overload and the erotic impact of driving 100 miles home will contribute to a profound sense of sexual deadness. As will watching too much TV once he arrives.

7 If his libido is completely flattened, there are several questions you should ask his doctor. What about a blood test? What about a thyroid check? If he's taking prescribed drugs, enquire about the known side-effects. Prozac, for instance, is good for premature ejaculation in small doses but 20–40mg will zap his sex-drive, according to New York sexologist Dr Helen Singer Kaplan. In a study done in 1995, 34 out of 80 male patients reported loss of sexual interest while taking a selected group of other antidepressants. The anti-hypertensives are also notorious for damaging sexual ability. Alcohol can also damage testosterone production as well as potency.

IF HIS LIBIDO IS STILL FALLING, WHAT CAN BE DONE?

1 Loads and loads. The key to sex-drive is in encouraging the testes to produce more free testosterone but the catch is that he cannot always take a simple supplement, pill or injection remedy. So encourage him to re-think his lifestyle and consciously choose a diet rich in meat, fish and (even) pumpkin seeds. Zinc is the problem. 'Each ejaculation can expend up to 5 milligrams of zinc, or one third of his daily allowance,' says Dr Sara Brewer, author of *Better Sex*, and zinc deficiency impacts on free testosterone production.

2 But don't think the answer, says Dr Riley, is having him pump his body full of synthetic testosterone. Only one man in ten who complains of reduced sexual desire actually has a low testosterone level. 'It's true,' he says, 'that free testosterone levels tend to fall with age but generally they stay within the normal range. Many with low testosterone levels continue to experience acceptable levels of sexual drive.' Extra testosterone, it appears, can trigger the growth of seed cancers in the prostate; high levels will cause the testes to shrink and instead of making him sexy, HRT could make him more aggressive. 'I personally wouldn't take it,' adds Riley – although other doctors disagree.

3 You can definitely exploit the power of pheromones across a crowded room. These aromatic chemicals are produced when bacteria break down the sweat in the body's hot spots. The recommendation, therefore, is not to let him be in too much of a rush to wash away (fresh) sweat. BO takes at least 24 hours to become socially offensive. Before that, BO is really sex musk. So is the scent of oral sex but if you really want a buzz then the underarm hair, seat of wonderful sweat glands, should never be neglected. Actress Julia Roberts is not alone in shaving less frequently in this area – as revealed by photos of a recent film premiere. And Napoleon Bonaparte was an understanding sexologist when he scribbled a note to the Empress Josephine: 'Home in three days; don't wash.' Josephine, knowing when she was well off, obeyed.

'I chalk up the growing popularity of male-to-female oral sex,' says sexologist Dr Robert Francoeur, 'to this increased exposure to pheromones.' There's a lot in this, agrees Dr Riley, because it works directly on the hypothalamus, the sex-drive centre in the brain. 'Equally important is making sex more thrilling with pleasures like cunnilingus. That makes you want more sex – and sooner not later.

4 Exercise can boost his endorphin levels but research shows that competitive sport does even more for the male libido. In one experiment, two sets of basketball teams, one all-male, one all-female, were tested for their testosterone levels before and after a game. The men experienced a huge surge of testosterone before the game and another one if they beat the opposition (but not if they lost). The women's levels, however, remained much the same. A similar experiment was conducted on male fans during the 1994 World Cup. The testosterone levels of supporters of the winning team rose by nearly 30 per cent overall. We're not suggesting you rush him to the basketball court every night before bedtime. But you might like to take advantage of his arousal after watching his team win on TV.

5 Sexually explicit videos can also help raise lost libido. In one experiment, when a group of selected couples were shown erotic films in the early afternoon, their lovemaking rates in the evening rose significantly. The effects tailed off only when the researchers ran out of new videos! This confirms some 70s research conducted by the National Sex Forum in San Francisco who used to hold the SAR (Sexual Attitude Restructuring) Weekends. Volunteers were asked to view over 40 sexually explicit films in a group setting over two full days. Afterwards, people could hardly walk straight; most reported a significant loss of sexual inhibition and many paired off into their private dormitories.

6 You could also try massaging his testicles. There is some anecdotal evidence that this increases testosterone production although the evidence is not very convincing. On the other hand, testicular massage definitely triggers the early phases of sexual arousal when prostatic fluid is moved down the urethra towards the penile tip. Done regularly, this will raise overall levels of desire.

7 Talking of raising things, Viagra, the impotence pill, is claimed by its makers to have no effect on sexual drive. Yet, since erection will be associated with arousal, it is quite likely in time to lead to arousal. Changes to colour vision experienced by some users confirm that Viagra does reach the brain. So perhaps this drug could have some minor aphrodisiac effect after all?

8 Help him to think positive. For those under-45, lifestyle rather than health is usually the problem. So take a pro-active approach, if his libido falters. When you both get tired, depressed, and your sex life isn't working or isn't working very well, you need a rest and a holiday. What he doesn't need is to go four hours' clubbing then back to your place for an attempt on the world endurance record. Remember, he can't spend the same energy twice.

FINALLY

ALL the research agrees that if he wants to retain his appetite for life, a 'healthy mind in a healthy body' is a slogan that works. Design-wise, male sexuality is fragile. So, if he overworks or overplays the system, he mustn't expect his sexuality to be overjoyed – survival comes first, before fun or even reproduction. Hormones do control much of sexual drive but not like a machine. His brain and emotions control his hormones. So when he 'goes off sex' he should think about *feelings* that have gone wrong as well as those potential chemical imbalances. And remember, says Dr Riley, there is no such thing as a scientifically proven aphrodisiac. 'If oysters worked, there wouldn't be one left in the ocean.'

the ART OF great sex

Don't feel embarrassed because by reading this book you're planning to improve your love-life. Hell, we're writing this book and we're *still* planning to improve our love-lives. As we've already emphasised, one of the tedious facts of sex is that it suffers from the law of diminishing returns. So more is less if you stick to the same routine. There's a famous memoir by the American model, Viva, written in the early 1970s and based on her experiment of staying in bed and making love for three days without stopping. On Day Three, she complains that she doesn't seem able to come any more. At the heart of this frustration lies a paradox. You'll *always* want what you can't have. Delayed gratification is sweetest. Question: what might you do to get the man of your dreams into bed? Answer: an awful lot more than you would to stimulate your available partner. That's a crying shame because novelty can begin at home.

THE SEVEN NIGHTS OF LOVE

So if you want to stir things up here's a game two lovers can play to harness the power of delayed gratification. It naturally depends on deferring most orgasmic sex until the final night.

PRELIMINARY

To get the ball rolling, toss this copy of *How to Make Great Love to a Man* across the bed and say 'What do you think of this?' or 'Would you like to improve your sexual health?' or 'Look at the fantastic massage you get on Day Two!' Alternatively, don't let him into the full secret but say you've been reading about body-mapping and would he like to go on a geography feel trip with you under the duvet?

DAY ONE

body-mapping: the secret gardens of delight

The best torturers conceivably make the best lovers. So with apprehensions high, the first scenario deliberately keeps the temperature a little cool. This also helps with any joint inhibitions.

After a good half bottle of wine each, roll the dice to see who goes first in the 'Sexological Exam'. The couple sit naked facing each other. The one who starts touches (non-genitally) the other person with a specific stroke and the recipient marks that touch for sensuality on a scale of Plus-3 to Minus-3. The strokes should be varied from super-gentle to quite strong. As the body is covered, a mental map of the most sensitive areas and the way they like to respond will be formed.

The partners may either take it in turns stroke by stroke, or do all their touching in one go then swap over. The aim should be to learn a secret about the partner's body – to find a four-inch square piece of non-genital flesh which you can drive wild. Or – you confirm your knowledge of your partner's favoured places. Even old-established lovers may have grown careless and sloppy here. The night ends (without sex) in tongue-kisses of the aforesaid four-inch square, a big hug and alcoholic serenity.

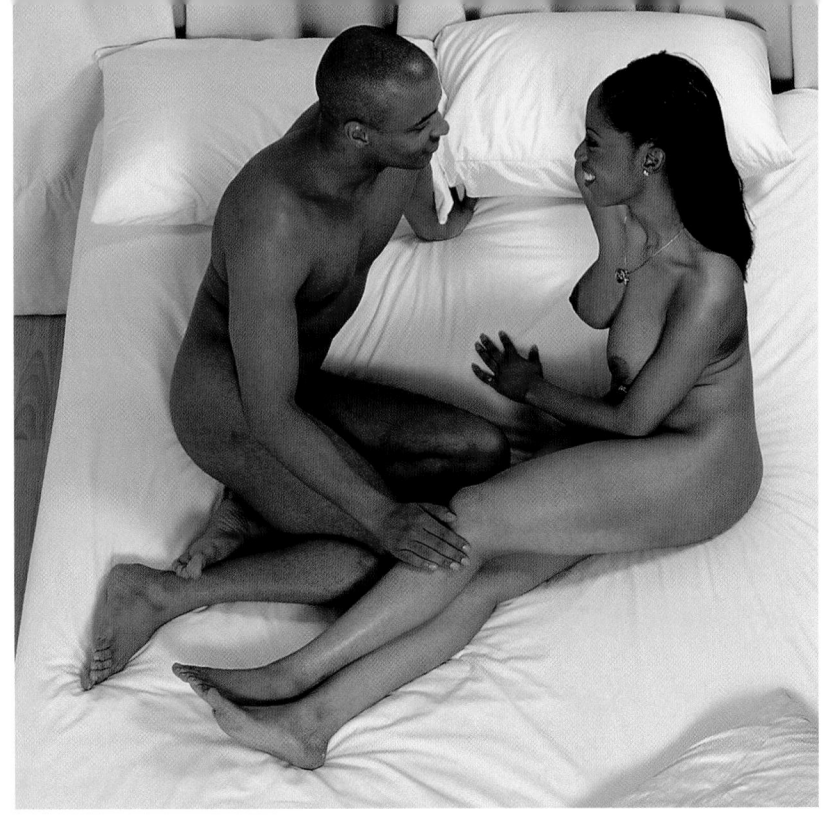

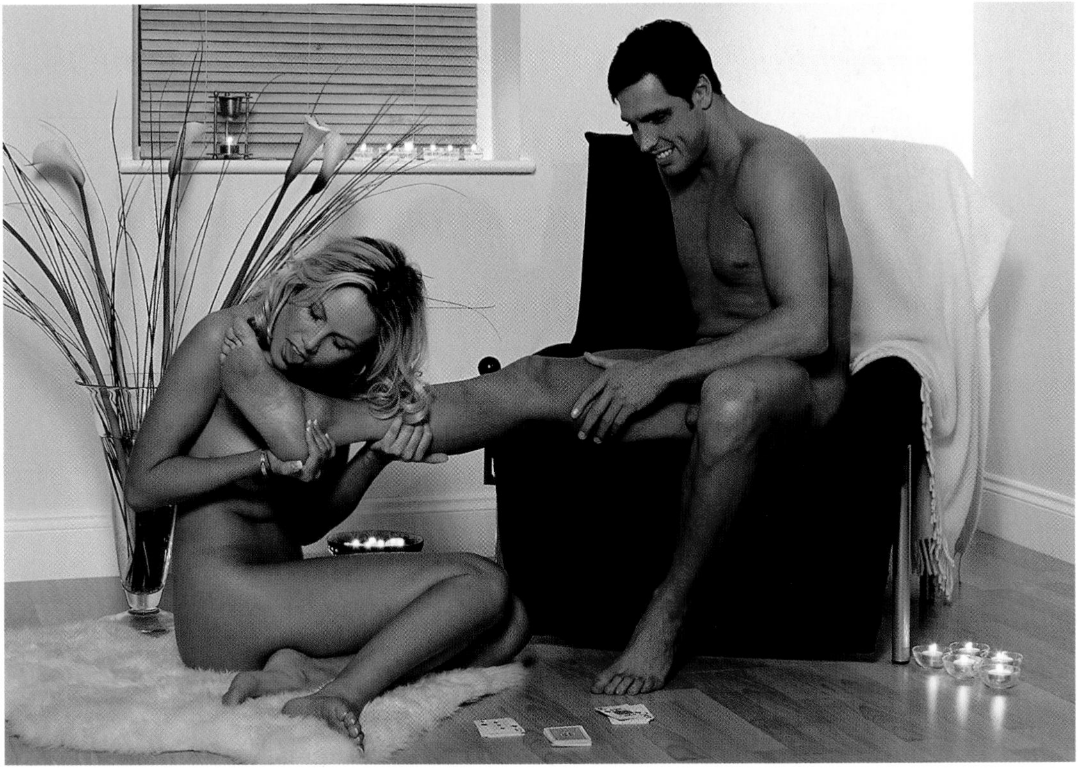

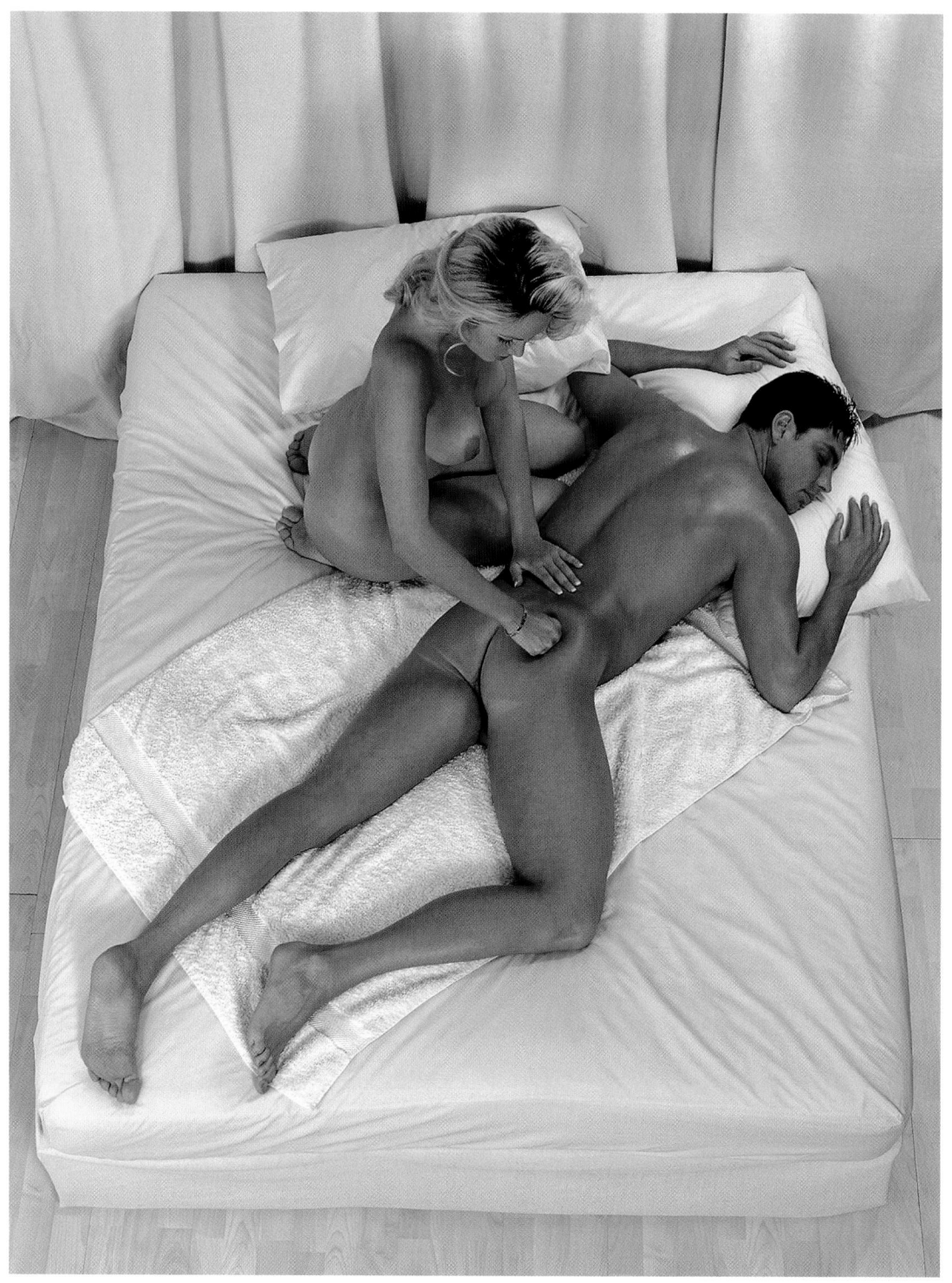

DAY TWO
sensual massage is the match of the day

Everyone loves this from small babies to oldies. Why? Because the skin as the largest organ of the human body enjoys a monopoly of nerve-endings. If you've *ever* been accused of rushing into intercourse in the past, now is your chance to compensate. Sensual massage is foreplay minus the sex. Therefore, your partner ends up wanting more. By happy accident, so do you. In the interests of our seven-day package, you steadfastly withhold.

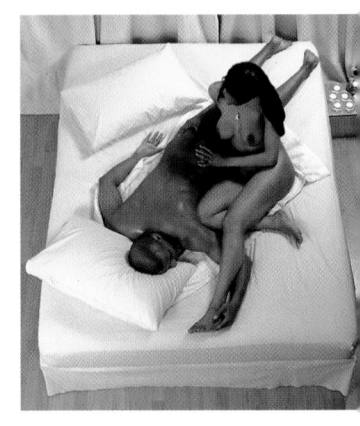

Remember to use warm hands, warm oil and play music he likes by candlelight. Start by massaging his back, keep your hands continuously on his flesh and push your strokes away from the heart. Brilliant spots to titillate include hands and feet, backs of knees, points of buttocks and any secret zones of passion discovered 24-hours previously.

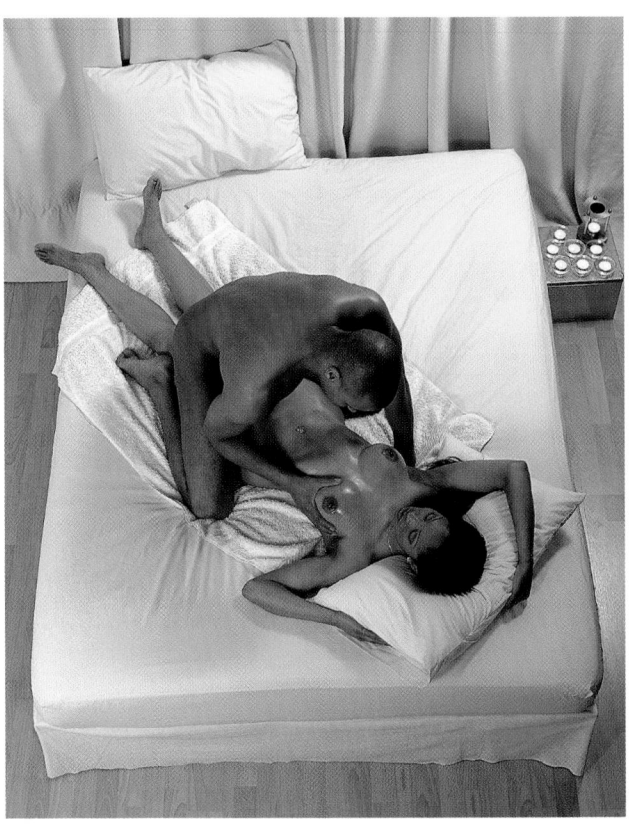

To take it further, use a special glove with fake fur on one side and velvet on the other (either make your own or buy one from a sex boutique). Feathers have been known to make grown spies confess to anything and ice cubes applied to earlobes or nipples will please those with a moderate interest in pain. If he's more masochistic, suggest that he wears a blindfold (miraculously, you have one) so that you can pretend he's your prisoner destined to suffer improper handling. Conclude by providing him with gentle balls-ache – you deliberately understroke the sides of the scrotum but steadfastly refuse to address the penis. If he complains, say that he can touch himself later on. Go easy on the verbal threats – just remember you're being massaged *next*.

DAY THREE
is about exploring your fantasies
Of course, some people have little sexual imagination. If you ask them
to recite a sexual fantasy they mutter the equivalent of 'Excuse me?'

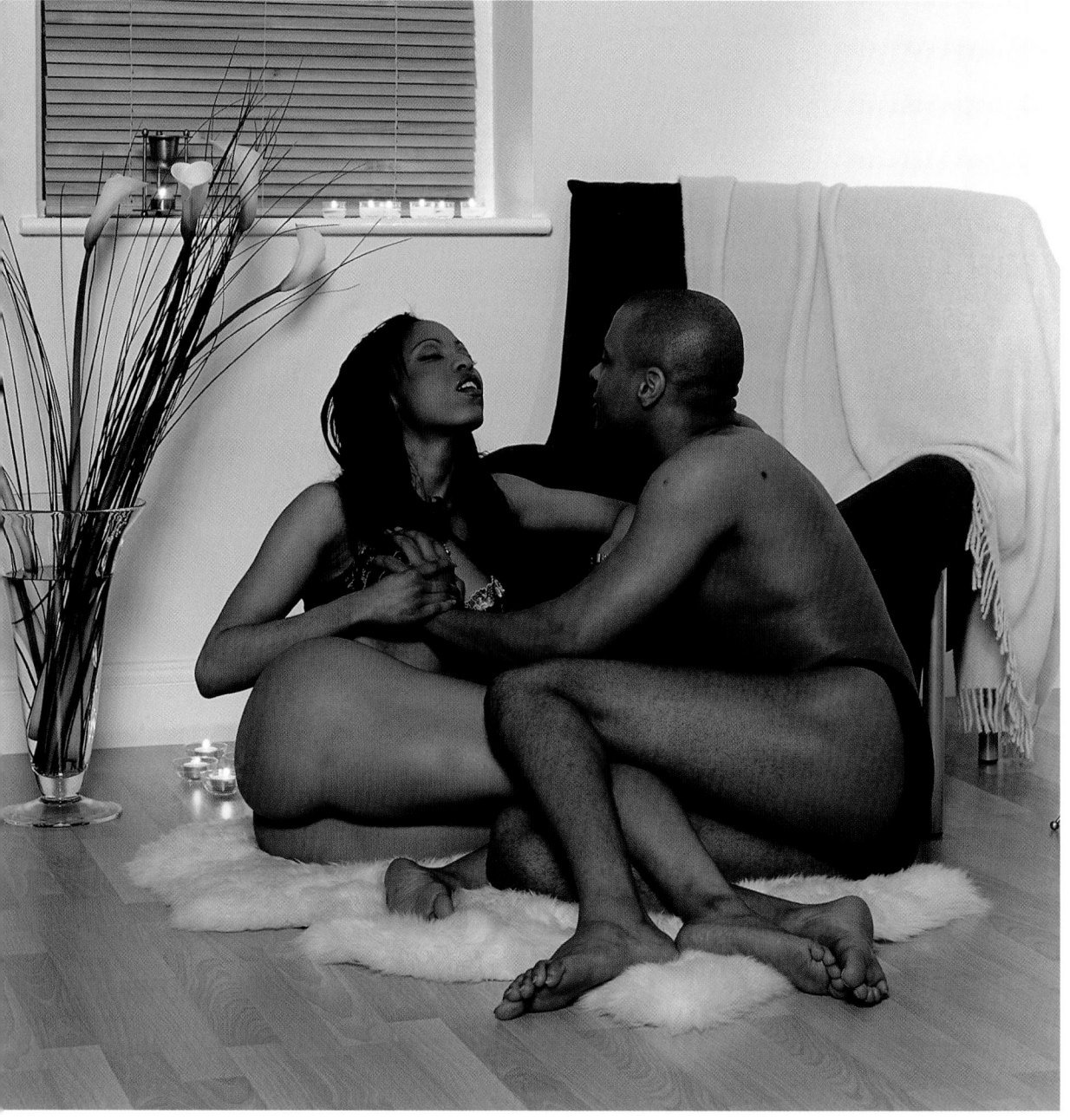

Sigmund Freud said, 'When two people make love there are at least four people present – the two doing it and the two they're thinking about.' But, leaving aside terrible thoughts of mum and dad, how can you use and generate better fantasy action?

Well, you could try confessing those secret wishes you know you've been harbouring for years. Come on – we've nearly all got something wonderful in our heads to be ashamed of. These fantasies will probably be politically incorrect to boot. But *his* favourite wank dramas are just as likely to feature dirty flirts as environmentally minded social workers. You could try reading Nancy Friday's book on sexual fantasies aloud, since men can respond to soft porn in words. But go carefully since some of these explicit stories were originally culled from the pages of men's magazines and written by men pretending to be women – 'I'm air hostess Sonja, founder of the Mile-High Club ... ' and you don't want to confuse his gender awareness too much.

Or to break the ice simply discuss which of the following you most fancy: Brad Pitt, Tom Cruise or Sean Connery (as he was in the 60s). You then enter into the technique called 'Guided Fantasy', building a sensual scenario in words. You might, for instance, start with a room, add some music, put in a four-poster, conjure up room-service, add personnel, create dialogue and bring on Rosa Kleb.

Alternatively, rent a video by Candida Royalle. These blue movies were specially created to be female-friendly with frame after frame of lustful longings across crowded restaurants and yards of compulsory snogging before a fastener gets zapped. But first, hand your lover the remote control with the instruction to pause the action whenever something happens on screen that he has *sometimes* secretly wished would happen to him. Afterwards, you make his video dreams come true – short of coital climax. We're still trying to last the full seven nights without anything disgusting like that.

If you possess a sense of humour, now's the time to consider toying with the gender roles. This won't be for everyone but some men get off on being decorated with your underclothes or adding a dash of colour to their lips ... Don't panic – it's only like dipping a toe into the *Rocky Horror Show* at home. Just remember to lock the doors and use a proprietory cosmetic removal agent before letting him bike to work next morning.

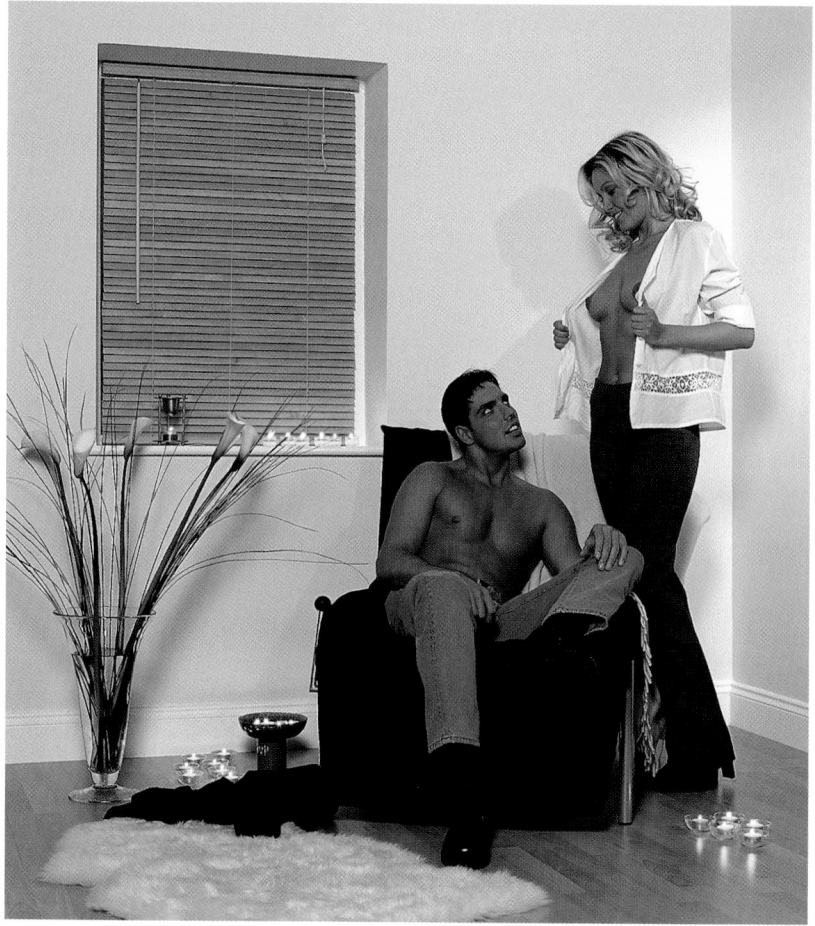

DAY FOUR
mind-mapping

Each person gets to ask up to five revealing questions and the other person undertakes to reply truthfully. The answers are designed to show or confirm whether your partner is really a risk-taker or a risk-hater, really patient or impulsive, really broad-minded or ultimately reserved. For example: would you ever make love in a lift, car, field, train, plane, office or on a beach? Have you ever done so? Describe. At the end of the evening, the dice is rolled and one person chooses whether to massage or be massaged. The catch is that the one massaged is also blindfolded while the other replays their favourite fantasy in teasing words. Again, no complete sexual act, though the massage may veer towards what one small boy has called the "rogerous" zones too.

DAY FIVE
who's in charge?

Both lie naked and by a cut of the cards take it in turns to be dominant for about one hour. Follow precisely the formula described in Chapter Nine – Games and Scenes to Make Men Weep For Joy.

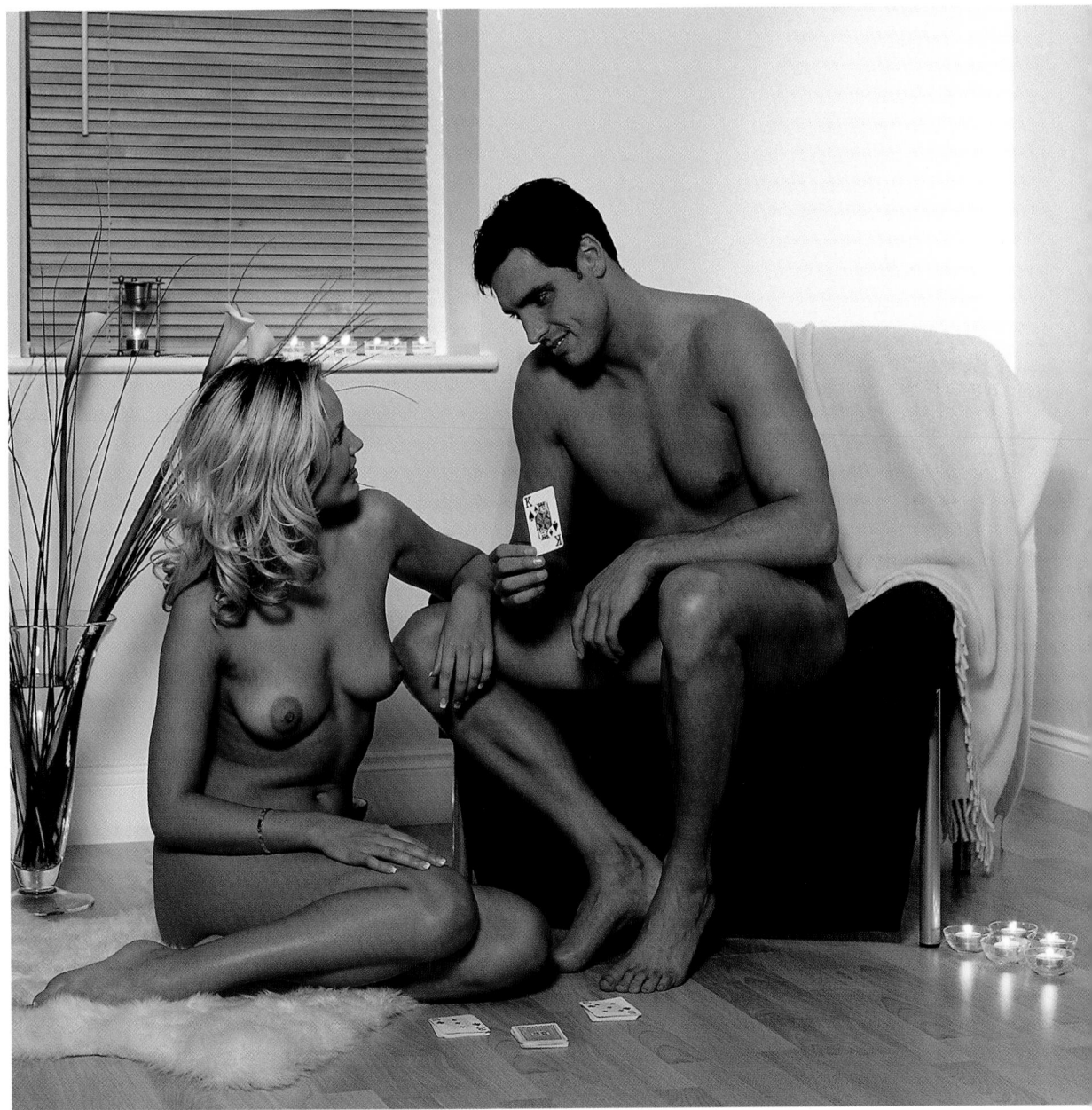

GIVING A GENITAL MASSAGE

Remember that you are not aiming at bringing him to orgasm although you can happily apply these techniques on another occasion to take him all the way. With more than 72,000 nerve endings, hands create and receive more stimulation than any other region apart from the genitals.

1 **The Lemon Squeezer** – Steady the penis by grasping it around the halfway mark with one hand. Then rub the cupped palm of your other hand over and around the head of the penis, as if you were juicing a lemon. It helps if you close your eyes and actually feel your hand brushing across the surface. Circle very gently moving your hand first ten times clockwise and then a further ten times anticlockwise. Use steady strokes rather than slow ones and, as you become adept at making them, you will find they take on a particular rhythm.

2 **The Corkscrew** – Put one hand on each side of the penis shaft. Slide your hands around in the opposite directions at the same times – as if you were trying to twist the penis in half (although you're not) and then slide them back again. Repeat ten times. It really goes without saying that you need to do this gently, but don't be afraid of maintaining quite firm pressure.

3 **Hand Over Hand** – Slide your cupped hand over the head and down the shaft. Before it goes to the base, bring the other hand up to the head to repeat the stroke. This is like the simple children's game of 'hand over hand', where you repeatedly bring your hand from underneath the pile of hands and place it on top, never breaking the rhythm. It has to be performed pretty quickly. The aim is to keep up a continuous hand-over-hand movement so that the head of the penis remains uncovered for as little time as possible.

4 **The Squeeze Technique** – Used to control ejaculation. If your partner tells you that he has the urge to come, grasp his penis and press your thumbs against it just below the glans (of head). Maintain firm pressure for a few seconds or until his desire to ejaculate has subsided. (You can also use your mouth – teeth covered by lips – to produce the same sharp 'nip'.)

5 **Togetherness** – Apply generous amounts of lubricant to both your and your partner's hands. Position your hands on either side of the penile shaft, palms facing each other, penis in the middle, fingers pointing towards his chin as if in prayer. Ask him to place his hands around yours and control the motion and speed of your palms. Terrific for non-verbal communication of exactly which touches he most enjoys.

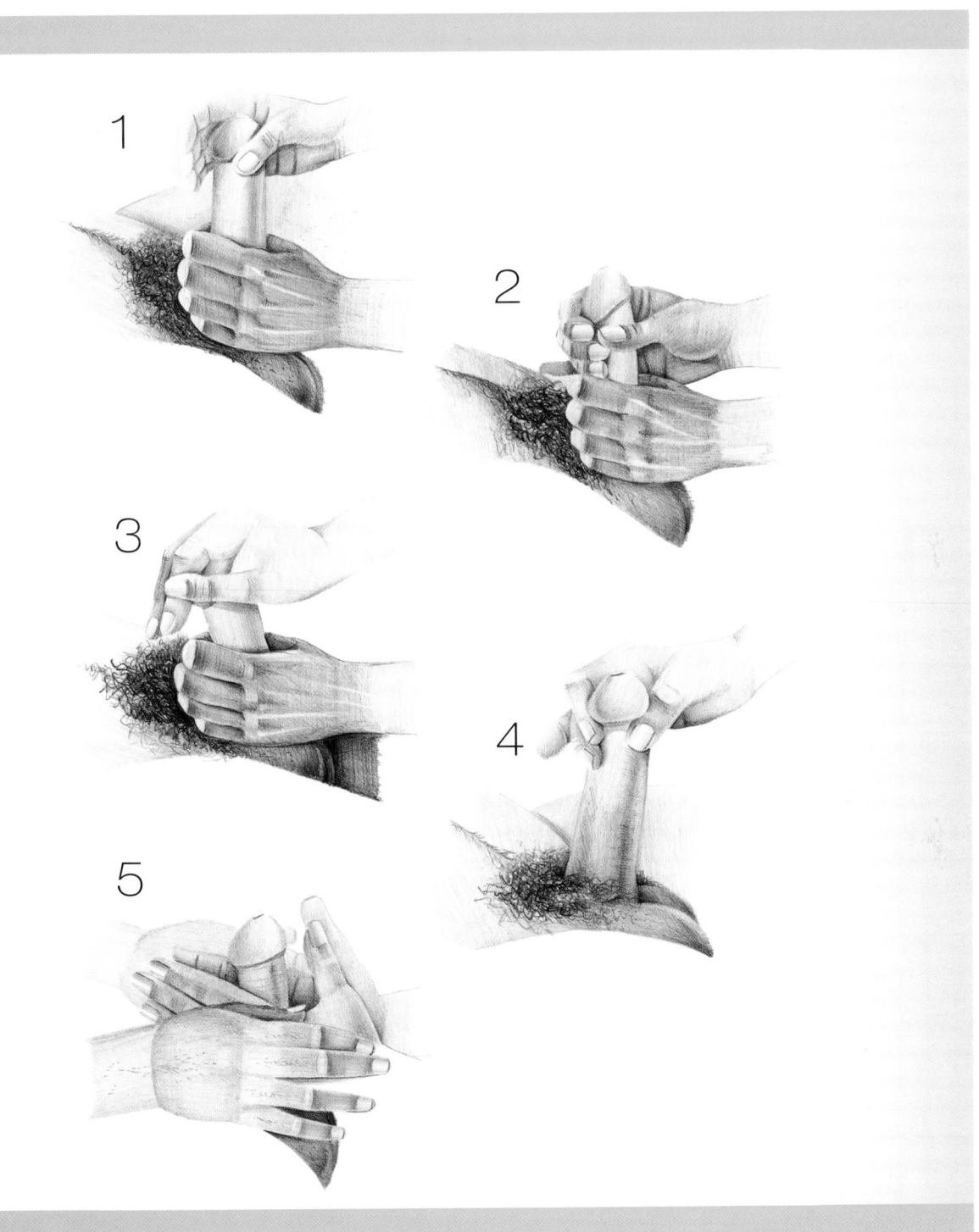

DAY SIX
coital alignment

After all that heady stuff, a quiet night of reflective anticipation. Since tomorrow is your new relationship's first grand prix, it's as well to get the sexual wheels aligned in advance. You wouldn't find Michael Schumacher roasting round the track without undertaking preliminary telemetry and it's the same with sex. Most intercourse, for instance, when practised by young people, fails to align the pubic bones. Result – his thrusts do little or nothing for her thrust receptors. You have two of these – one situated in the clitoris, the other inside the anterior wall of the vagina (if you're lucky enough to own the G-spot model). Some women can only

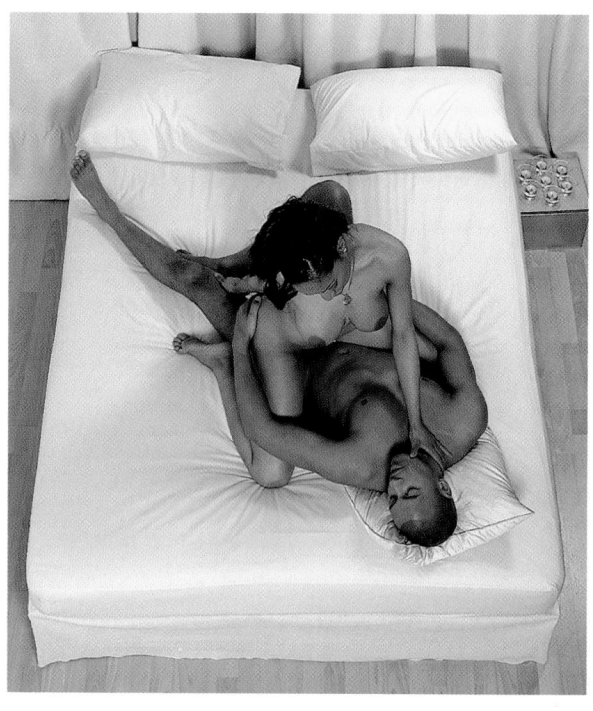

climax in the 'woman on top position'. Some men cannot come in the 'woman on top' position. There is clearly enormous scope for disappointment and as a couple you should now lie side by side and explore which strokes do most for your reproductive organs and which positions you would ideally receive if lucky enough to gain first place on the grid tomorrow. The catch is this – you must *now* do a dress-rehearsal. Yes, you try out your favourite positions and match movements to wishes but keep your underclothes on. Orgasms optional.

DAY SEVEN

By now you should be bursting with desire. We've arrived at where we've been leading. Shake of the dice – and the winner (this week) gets the sex of their dreams. The loser gets great sex but remains hungry for just that little bit extra ...

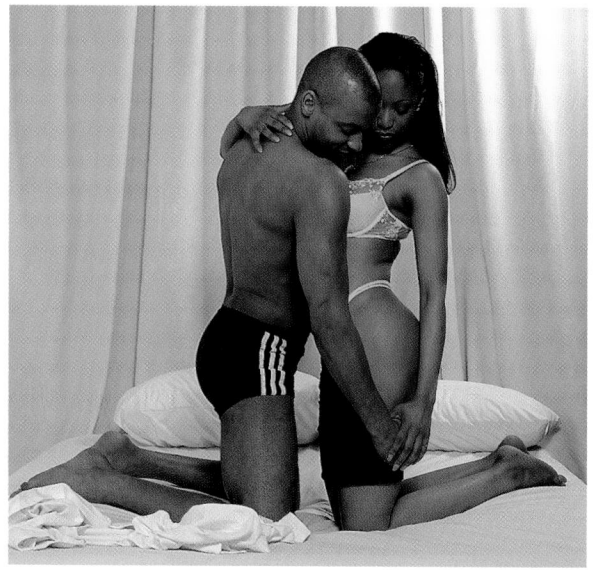

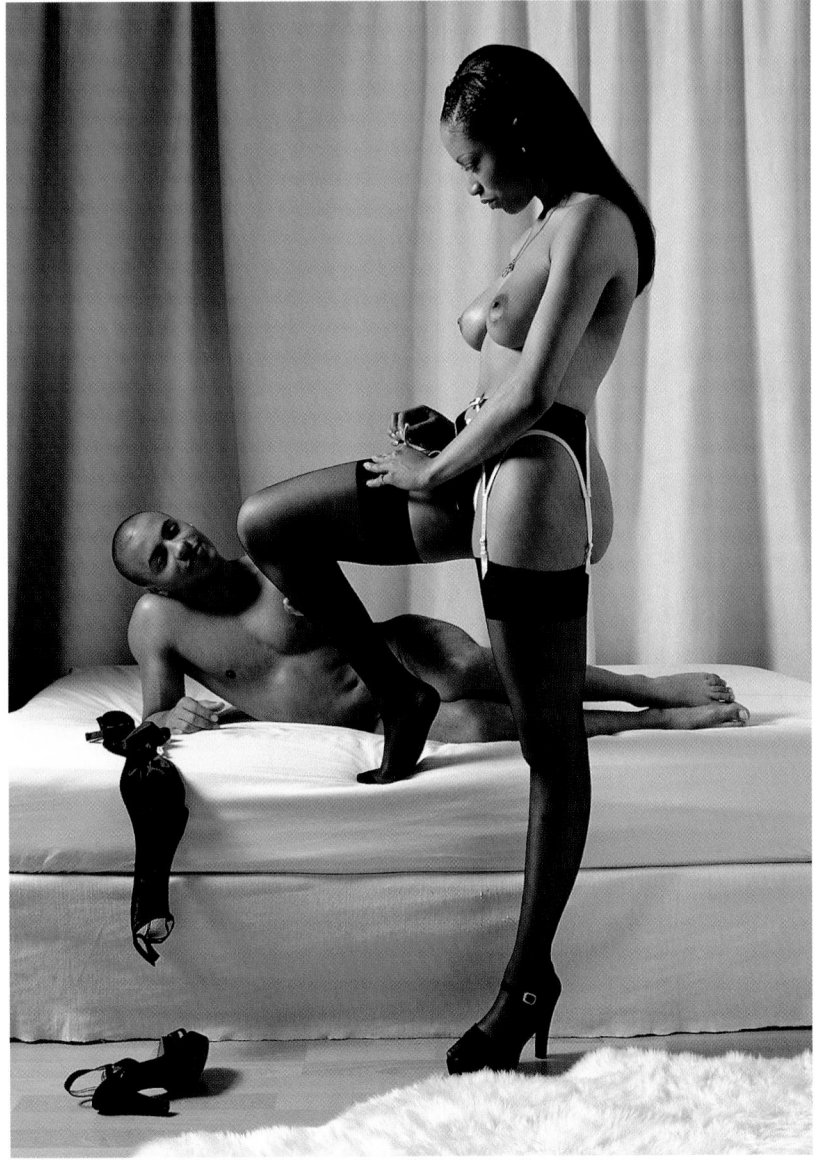

Of course, games-playing sometimes leads to tears. Winning and losing are very important experiences in childhood and grown-ups frequently feel overwhelmed by unpleasant sibling-style sensations. Competition in bed is not always erotically productive.

To give you a slight edge, however, here are some of the hidden codes you might like to make use of when dealing with your man in the preliminaries of passion.

EIGHT SEXUAL SECRETS MEN DON'T WANT YOU TO KNOW

There is some truth in the notion that men tell their mistresses and ladies of pleasure what they want in bed but their wives and girlfriends what they think they ought to hear. Jokes abound – what's undersized and hairless and thinks it's Antonio Banderas? Or what's strong and silent and yearns to be dressed in pink and lace? Or what's both Dr Jekyll and Mr Hyde. You've guessed the answer – it's a man.

Of course, if you're trying to probe secrets, the fact that most men are uncomfortable with emotional disclosure presents a difficulty. Actor Dennis Waterman speaks for many in the silent-male majority: 'I'm not very good at relationship-type conversations. I find this whole idea of "we must talk about things" doesn't help very much, it wastes time and is often destructive. I'm a bit of a coward and I don't like talking terribly person-ally. I keep things to myself. If I've got a problem, it's mine. I don't want to change that. I'm over 40 and it's too late to change anything really.'

What Dennis Waterman is saying on behalf of those he represents, however, is that if he experiences any personal emotional difficulties that do not get automatically resolved, then nothing gets resolved at all. On the subject of sex, men are still full of advertising, fantasy and denial with the issue approached from the point of view of their potential achievements rather than rational human intimacy. However, you have to cope with men as they are rather than how you would like them to be and a wealth of evidence suggests that the attempt is worthwhile. Statistics on divorce and health show that men need your intimacy even though they won't always say so. When it works, they become far better at loving you back. So here's a list of the primary male codes. Remember that generalisations are fallible but that's no reason to be afraid of them:

MEN LIKE SEXUAL CONTROL

Even the chap who fancies being 'submissive' wants to choose when! For other men saying 'I love you' is not a simple expression of delight in wife or partner, it often represents emotional defeat: 'Damn, I've put myself at risk of rejection again.' Men's solution to this problem is to experience sex as a separate entity, which is why they might talk of 'my

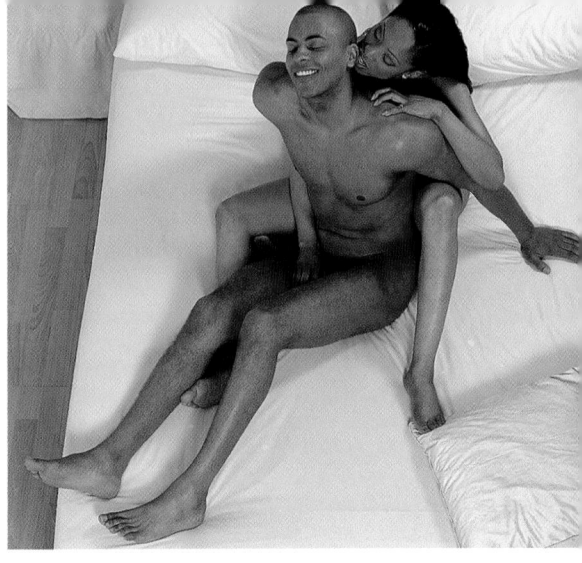

sex life' as if it happens almost by itself: 'I didn't fancy her but decided to give it a go to keep myself up to scratch... ,' one man wrote. 'I can't function if the sexual decisions are ever in the woman's hands' (*Executive Magazine*, April 1982).

advice: Forewarned is forearmed. Find out carefully about his favourite ways to be approached. If he does appear wary of closeness, give him time to realise how trustworthy you've always been – in fact, the one who really looks after him. Whatever else, men respect loyalty.

MEN SUFFER FROM PENIS ENVY

Men don't always let on, but are desperate for women to find them visually... impressive. Men believe women are fascinated by what's up front; in fact, research shows women are more typically observing men's behinds. 'He's got some nice jeans that aren't too tight but show off his bum – my favourite part of his body – nicely,' (singer Gloria Estefan on husband Emilio). Whatever Freud said, it's not women who want to look like stallions but men who are preoccupied with how their sexual appearance compares to others. As a result, the 'executive organ' gets idealised into a machine, tool or rock of unbelievable durability. In fact,

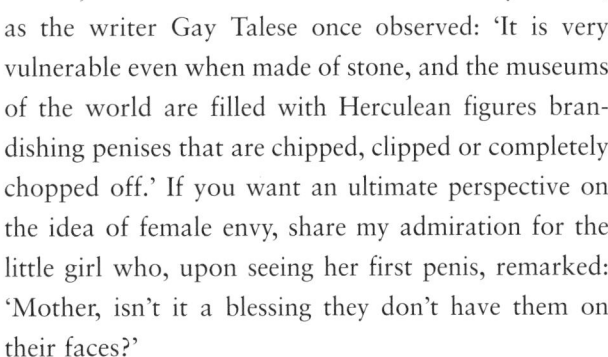

as the writer Gay Talese once observed: 'It is very vulnerable even when made of stone, and the museums of the world are filled with Herculean figures brandishing penises that are chipped, clipped or completely chopped off.' If you want an ultimate perspective on the idea of female envy, share my admiration for the little girl who, upon seeing her first penis, remarked: 'Mother, isn't it a blessing they don't have them on their faces?'

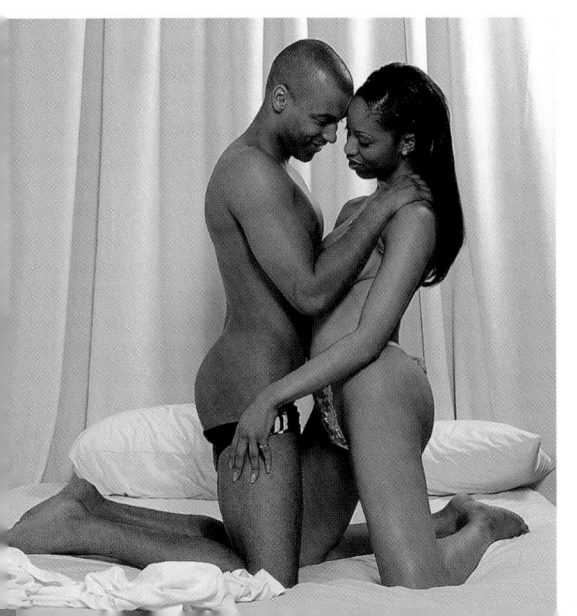

advice: even if it is not your favourite bodily item, never disparage his manly proportions. If you actually are 'impressed', say so, with fervour.

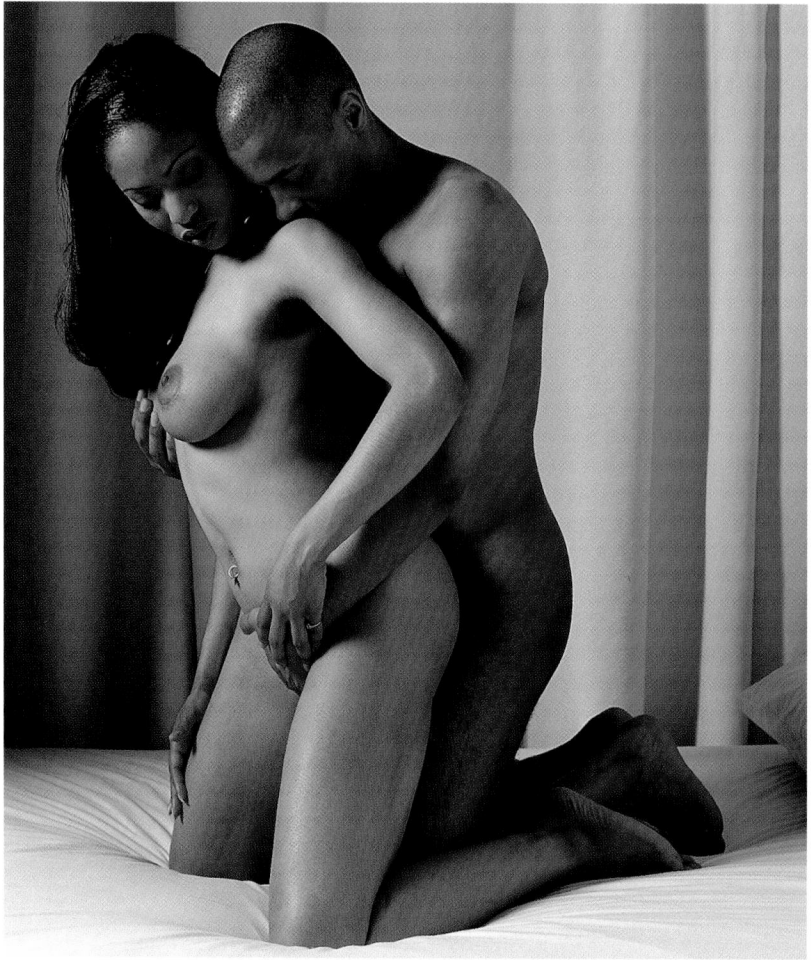

MEN HATE SEXUAL CRITICISM

Only male masochists like you to mention the shortcomings of their sexual technique or performance. George and Carol came for counselling after she had complained that he 'went at it like I was a roll of old carpet, he was hopeless'. Carol was asked how she phrased her complaint? 'Just like that,' came the puzzled response. 'He was hopeless so I told him.' Naturally enough, something inside George gave up hope with Carol and it was hardly surprising that he subsequently became impotent.

advice: If you want him to alter his behaviour in bed, learn to use positive language, not 'I can't stand it when you do X ...' but 'It's really wonderful when you do Y ... and I'd love you do some more of it right now, please.' Remember, most of us were naive lovers when we began.

MEN WANT WOMEN TO CLIMAX

Whatever they say, most men take credit if a woman responds orgasmically to them and feel both responsible and miserable if she doesn't. This is true regardless – regardless of her history and his level of skill. For instance, Geoff's ego was crushed when Evie didn't come to his star performance. She explained that what had happened with her uncle when she was a teenager still gave her sexual nightmares. Geoff couldn't begin to see what this had to do with him. As he put it: 'Every other girl told me I was a great lover. Now it suddenly disappears!' Or take the case of Lynne, quoted in the Kramers' book *Why Men Don't Get Enough Sex* (Virgin): 'We'd been having sex for six years so you think he'd get it right by now. If I don't have an orgasm, that injures his pride, so I fake it to keep him happy.'

advice: You are the expert on how your body works and no man can make you enjoy yourself unless you decide to let go. Nor can he give you the pleasure you crave unless you find a way to show him how. Faking, we stress, is always a mistake – it only trains a man *not* to satisfy you. If you convey the idea that all is wonderful when it isn't, your partner can only be expected to repeat his mistakes permanently. So, understand he needs to feel appreciated but help him to get it right. Show him how to create moods and fantasies, where to touch and when to be gentle and when to abandon control.

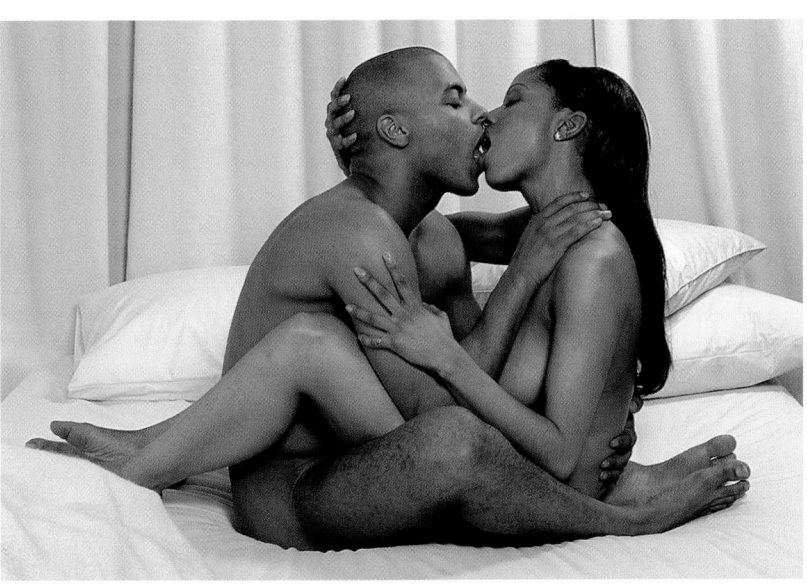

MEN LIKE PORNOGRAPHY

Whatever they say, most men will watch pornography because it excites them. Most men will also look at short skirts, indiscreetly revealed bosoms and blatant visual signals from wet lips to wriggling bottoms. In fact, men's eyes zero in on the erogenous zones before their brains have had time to think. Women do the same, of course, but less openly and less often. The real issue here is not sexual politics but consideration for each other's feelings. Diana, for example, simply hated the way husband Brian leered at her girlfriends. She said he didn't just have a roving eye, it was practically revolving. When he started bringing home copies of sex videos, she threw an all-time wobbly. He was amazed. They survived the episode by agreeing to widen their views and modify their conduct – he would be more discreet; she would be more broad-minded. For Christmas, she bought him a Japanese *Pillow Book*. He gave her an eternity ring attached to a card that said 'I promise only to smile at strangers'.

advice: men may be basic, but window-shopping isn't an inevitable prelude to infidelity.

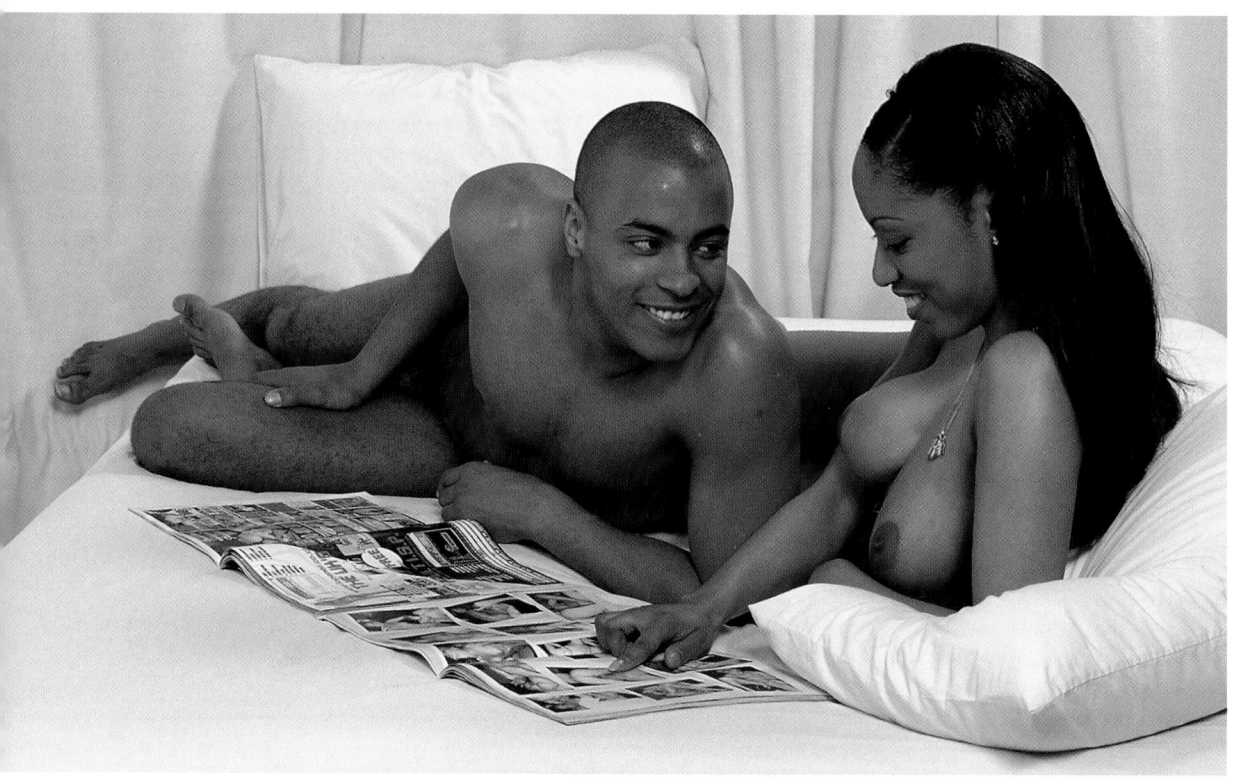

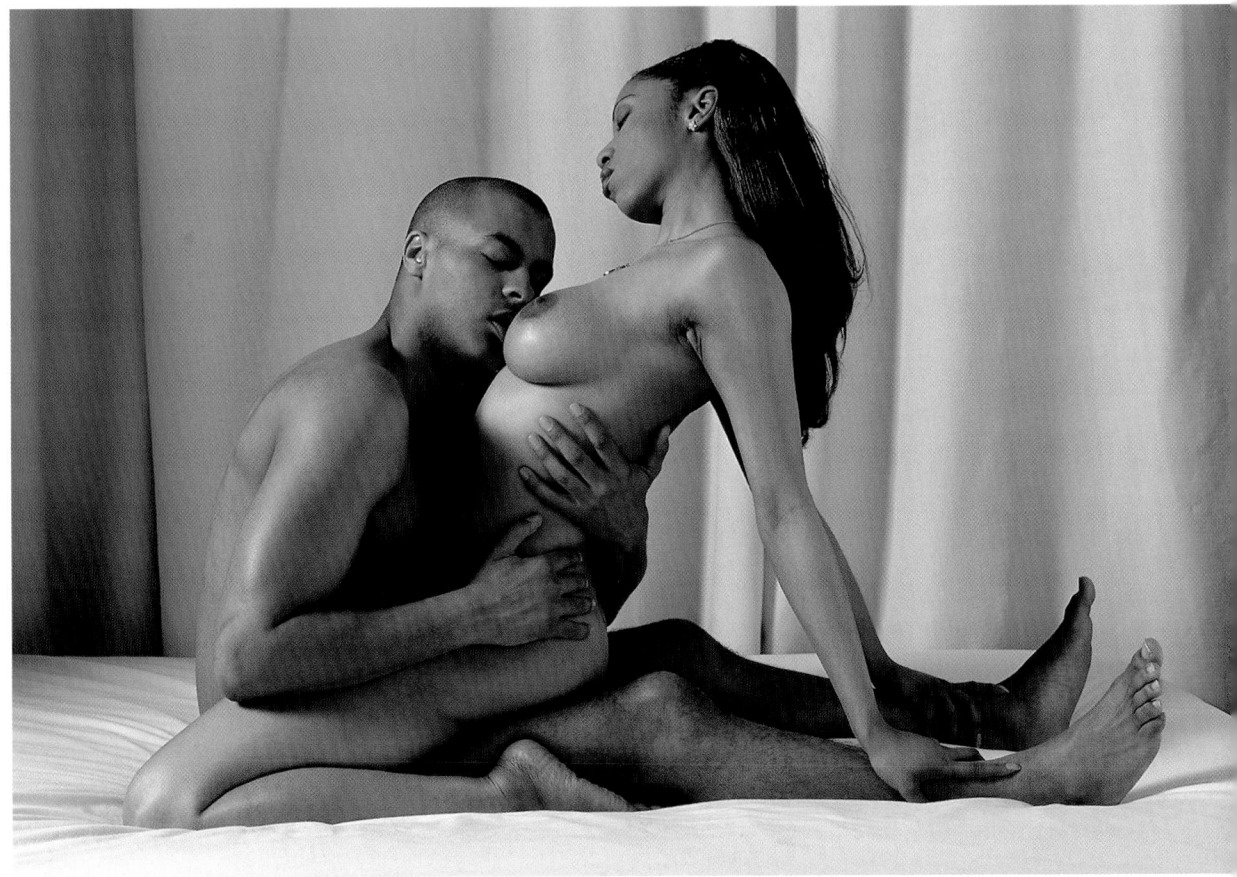

MEN ARE SEXUALLY SQUEAMISH

Some heterosexual men do not like everything about womanliness and cope poorly with the facts of menstruation, sexual odour and childbirth. They may never have been educated to understand these feminine essentials which therefore remain 'mysteries'. One of our correspondents, George B., for example, was shocked to his socks when he discovered that Mrs B. found breast-feeding a turn-on. It took a little persuasion to get him to see that breasts that are functional for a baby can stay 'sexy' for the parents. On the other hand, equally masculine men revel in sexual intimacy, especially a woman's secret scent.

advice: Tastes will always vary. If he has a problem, accept it at the outset but make sure he begins to learn how your body really works from month to month. A lot of male fastidiousness is really based on ignorance.

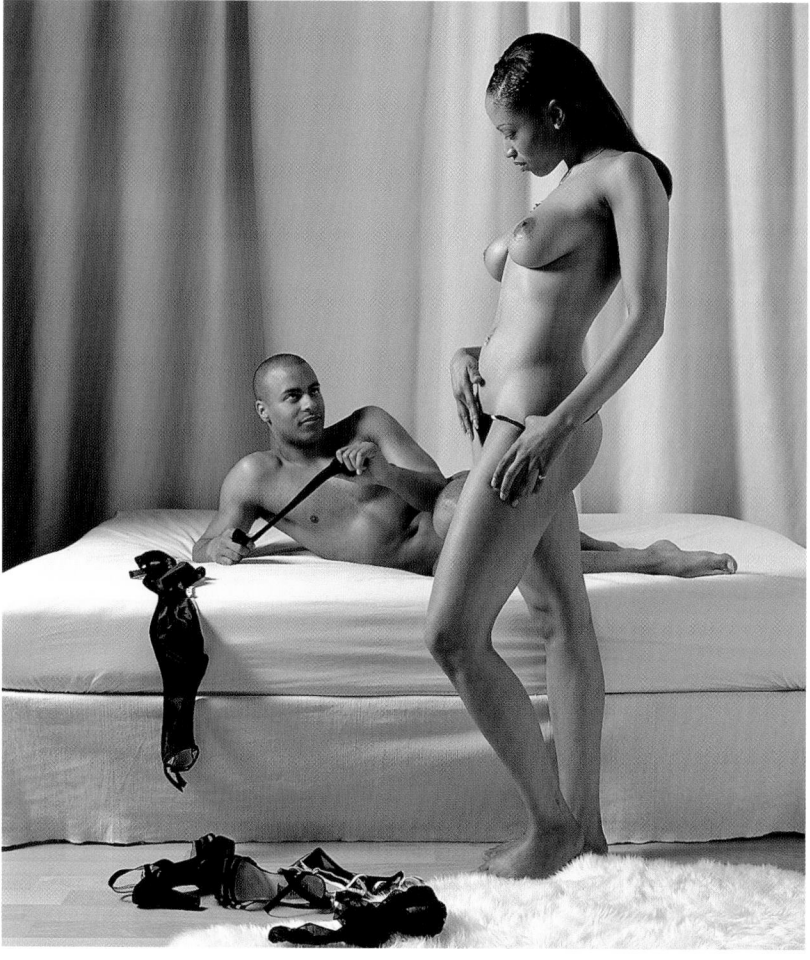

MEN ALWAYS HAVE SECRET FANTASIES

Most men have fantasies or near-fetishes of which they are ashamed or about which they feel embarrassed. One reason why many men are 'comfortable' with the idea of prostitution is that bold sexual commerce removes the awkwardness. Experienced working women expect men to 'have their little peculiarities'. During love-making, most men (like some women) will fantasise about others.

advice: Remind yourself that fantasy isn't reality – we no more get to choose which ones are exciting than we get to choose what we dream when asleep. It isn't a personal insult that someone's sexual imagination roams in bed. On the other hand, how could you use his 'little peculiar-ity' to your advantage? Perhaps tell him a story while he closes his eyes?

and finally ...

MEN AREN'T ALL SEX-MAD

It is not true that men will make love with you more often if you offer them sex more frequently. They will only pretend this is so. In fact, just as many men as woman have the headaches and just as many men as women withhold sex as a means of punishing or controlling their partners. The secret is this: men sometimes do not want to make love. After the age of 30, men also need more stimulation in order to be able to make love at all. June was extremely surprised, for instance, when the mere presence of her half-clothed body did not drive new boyfriend, 41-year-old Marcus, into a sexual frenzy.

advice: Don't be misled by male propaganda that they are ever-ready. But if you can tap into his fantasies, half your battle will be over – and the rest is down to deftness of touch.

A COMMON QUESTION

Q My boyfriend is always badgering me to have sex even when I only want a cuddle. Are men incapable of enjoying affection for its own sake?

A No, but they need guidance. Show your man these comments from remodelled males. From a doctor: 'Five minutes naked cuddle at the end of a bad day is worth more to me than an hour's verbal reassurance.' And from a stockbroker: 'Caressing my wife, even when that's all it amounts to, reinforces our love for each other, gives me confidence that she still loves me for what I am. It is a powerful antidote to business pressure, and better than a sleeping pill.' And an ex-manual worker: 'It took a crisis for my wife and me to learn the pleasures and comfort of skin-to-skin contact. Nothing eased the pain of losing my job so much as being together in that very close but special way.'

Offer your partner this deal: suggest you spend one evening together where you get as close as possible, removing all clothes and inhibitions, lying affectionately in each other's arms, for at least an hour, stroking and talking, even falling asleep. In return, the next night you might suggest having sex quickly and lustfully even without fully undressing – and don't condemn it if you haven't tried it. The secret of life (and sex) is a rhythmic balance between opposites. Further, therapist Barbara De Angelis says: 'There is a certain kind of spontaneity, surrender, and passion that men experience when they allow themselves just to have sex with a woman, which is often lost in a more conscious, slow, step-by-step lovemaking process.'

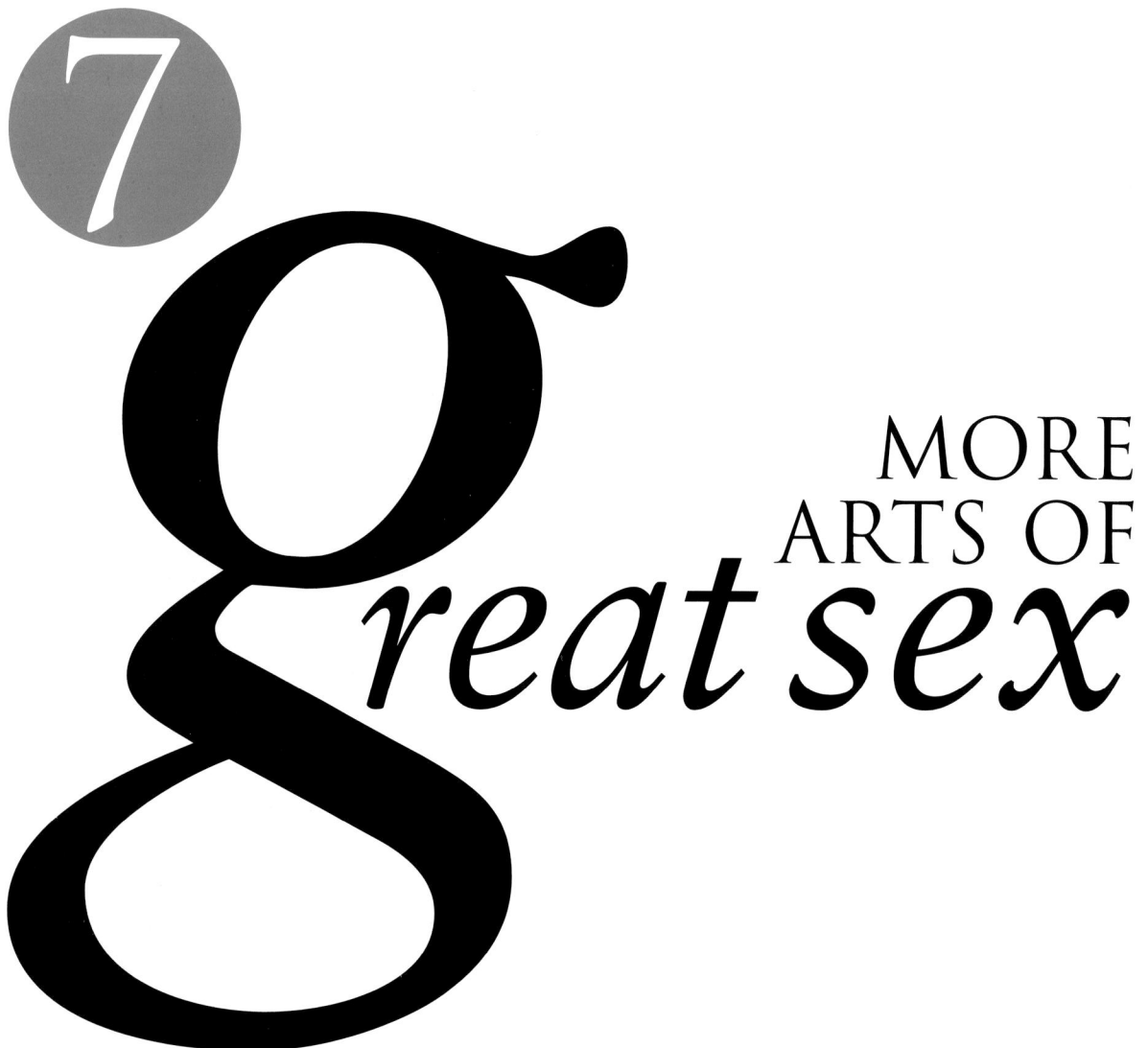

7

MORE ARTS OF great sex

HOW MEN FEEL ABOUT THEIR PRIVATE SEXUALITY

In this chapter, we look in more detail at a man's true sexual nature. Being able to offer the requisite arts of love means growing more aware of his behavioural sexual triggers. One way to understand what men want from their love-lives is to understand what they already obtain from sex by themselves.

Masturbation has always been somewhat emotionally and socially controversial. Irish playwright George Bernard Shaw is rumoured to have said: '99 per cent of people masturbate and one per cent are liars'. Several experts have challenged his figures. Others have argued that men do it more than women – because 'the male genitals come to hand more

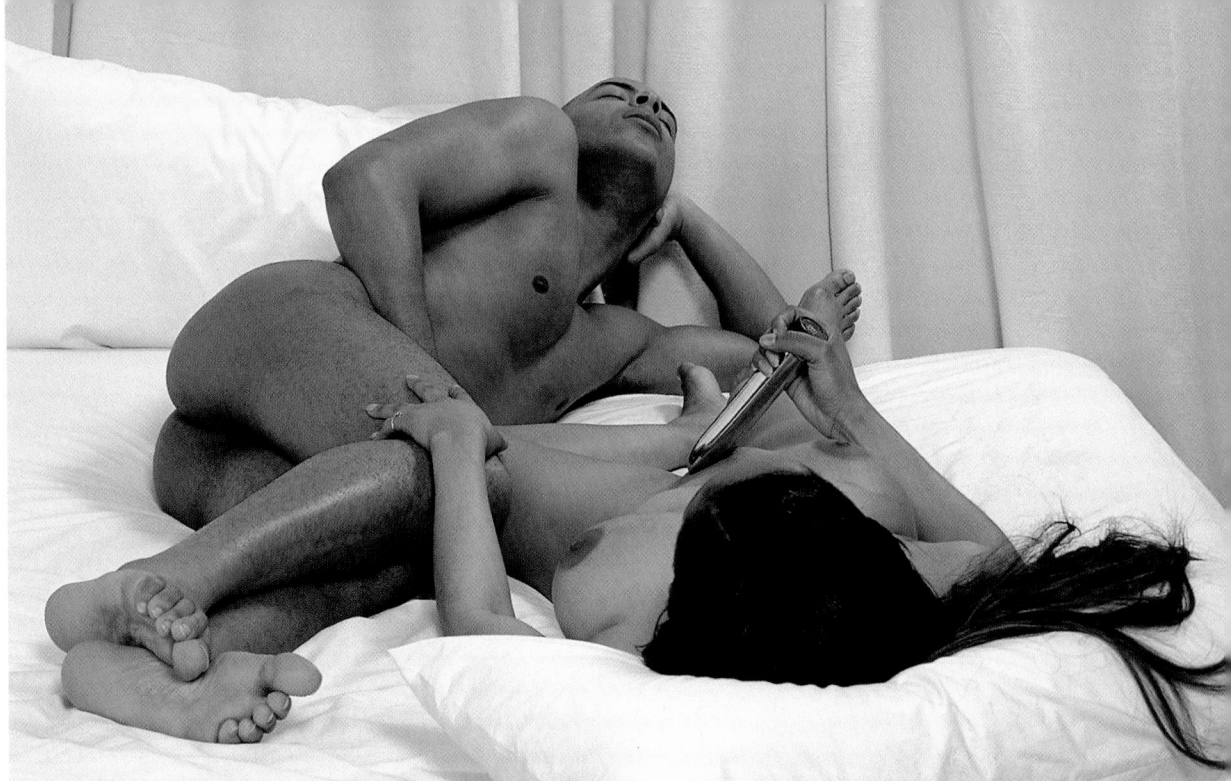

easily'. Feminists have responded that it's just as natural to put fingers *into* genitals as *around* them. And so the argument rages on.

What's really striking about Shaw's comment is the *positive* image it offers of masturbation. For most of the past 150 years, solo sex has had a bad press. The Victorians invented metal contraptions to stop children touching themselves at night. In the 1920s, popular European magazines like *Health and Strength* ran columns exhorting young men to renounce this 'vice' if they wished to prevent curvature of the spine and loss of cerebral fluid. In the 1980s, you could find fitness gurus urging avoidance of masturbation on the grounds that 'unnecessary orgasm' leaches the body of essential vitamins and minerals. And even today it is difficult to get reliable statistics on masturbation because 'discussion of this practice has met both with distaste and embarrassment from respondents ... and has therefore been excluded from our questionnaire' (a weighty book called *Sexual Attitudes and Lifestyles*, Penguin, New York, 1994).

HEALTH RISK IS ZERO

Yet few mainstream Western physicians or sexual experts would now actively condemn masturbation. After all, there is no major physical difference between an orgasm produced by hand or by intercourse.

Masturbation cannot cause blindness, weaken bones or make hair grow on fingers. These are old wives' tales. The practice has one basic purpose – pleasure. Side-effects include helping people become comfortable with their libido. It's a drug-free way to promote sleep. And if as seems likely everyone masturbates, at least a few times a year, it's hard to see how the activity could be labelled biologically unnatural.

PATTERNS OF MASTURBATION

Obstetrician William Masters used to joke with himself: 'Can I get the cord cut before the kid has an erection?' Infant boys play with their genitals from birth onwards as a means of seeking comfort. Full of pleasurable nerve-endings, the penis does not produce a proper orgasm prior to puberty. After puberty, male masturbation rates rocket. The purpose is now ejaculation. By early teenage, it's common to find males masturbating to orgasm up to 20 or 30 times a week (besides fondling themselves at other times). This pattern may decline in the 20s to about once a day but masturbation on a regular basis persists into middle age regardless of outside relationships.

Teenage masturbation results partly from innate desire and partly in response to social triggers. The latter include sexual media like *Penthouse* and *Playboy*, or Web sites with names like *The Erotic Strip* and *Ultracore.Com*. Boys tend to experiment with a wide range of masturbatory styles. Some may discover orgasm all by themselves in a 'wet daydream'. Some may play games with friends (of either sex) leading to orgasm. Many try to increase their sexual pleasure through a wide range of experimentation with time, place and circumstances.

HOW MEN DO IT

For example, a teenage boy may vary his routine by holding his hand still and moving his body. Some males, by contrast, do it 'standing up'. Sometimes, auto-fellatio is attempted, although this requires profound spinal flexibility. Items of underwear and handkerchiefs may be used to wrap or mop the penis. Masturbation may take place in any room at any time – the bathroom is a favourite locale; so is bed. Young male drivers have been known to masturbate while cruising the freeway – combining the love of sex with danger. Others use the telephone – to talk dirty with friends or commercial services.

MASTURBATION AND FANTASY

Most commonly men will look at a special selection of pictures or images to bring themselves into the right frame of mind to achieve orgasm. Sometimes, the masturbation session will commence with media, which are then ignored as passion takes hold. The man may keep his eyes closed relying entirely on his fantasies to take him 'over the edge'.

All the survey information seems to emphasise that men are more stimulated into sex by visual materials than women. It would be rare to find a man who does not use a favourite set of fantasies, thoughts or scenarios to accompany his self-stimulation. Eventually, a stock pattern becomes predominant. Usually this will be in accord with a man's basic sexual outlook. It would be strange, for instance, to find a heterosexual man lusting in his mind after images of gay sex. But it is not unknown for the 'power of the forbidden' to provide erotic excitement and men still appear to indulge in more deviant image-building than women.

Masturbation is by definition a rewarding activity. By having a lot of sex with themselves, males tend to mould their sexualities into an even more precise pattern of triggers. If a boy accidentally catches sight of his sister having sex, for example, masturbating repeatedly to the memory, he may well develop a taste for voyeurism in later life. If he comes into contact with his mother's more exotic underwear and incorporates the garments into his private sex routines or handles the materials while excited, it's possible he'll develop a range of adult fetishes. So masturbation plays a pretty important role in developing a man's individual sexual preferences.

How men feel about masturbation will vary. Some are obsessed with it – a small minority prefers 'DIY' sex to any other form. Most men would be embarrassed to be 'caught' masturbating by their partners, even the ones who would be happy to enjoy mutual masturbation with them in bed as a sexual variation. The male competitive instinct reserves a term like 'wanker" (masturbator) as one of abuse. The phrase 'go home and play with yourself' is a ritual dismissal of any inferior who is seen to be a failure in competing for the favours of mature females. But in their heart of hearts, most men know that masturbation is a sturdy standby when all else fails. It can do you no harm. You carry your own equipment around with you. It keeps men off the streets and out of trouble. Woody Allen wasn't far off the mark when he said that masturbation was sex 'with someone you love'.

THE JOYS OF MALE ORGASM

Naturally, most male masturbation is relentlessly focused on orgasm. The very idea of having solo sex without climax is somewhat preposterous. Yet it's said that orgasm isn't the only pinnacle of sex – the journey can be as much fun as the arrival. Nor do all male orgasms feel the same. In Chapter Four, we looked at ways to improve overall quantity. Here we take some time to look at how you can make your man's orgasm feel more profound.

ORGASM

To re-cap on the basics: an orgasm has been described as a body spasm akin to a sneeze. Tickle the right nerve and he must come. It is actually a physiological reflex that occurs when the correct sequence of thoughts and touches becomes synchronised with his personal arousal pattern. It may be an all-over body response, felt throughout the pelvis or solely focused on the penis, perineum and prostate. Some men talk of overlapping excitement in their breasts or even their heads. Some men report a profound post-coital headache. Some men feel as though their testicles are being stretched and report pain in that zone. Most men know the bitter-sweet discomfort of coming after being denied the opportunity for several hours. Orgasm will feel different on different occasions and at different ages and depending on whether a man is alone or in company. Mood controls orgasmic experience; so do emotions like love, joy and guilt.

WHAT ACTUALLY HAPPENS DURING CLIMAX?

Perhaps one of the most ignored features of climax is that, as soon as the responses begin, the brain temporarily loses control and places him into a timeless state. But the main part of the orgasm consists of rhythmic contractions at approximately 0.8 second intervals mediated via the penis. The biological purpose of orgasm is, of course, pregnancy, which is why male infertility is less common than feelings of low sensation or disappointing climax. Nature is more interested in ensuring the perpetuation of the species than in giving anyone a good time!

As we noted in Chapter Four, ejaculation appears to be a three-stage process. After arousal, a small bead of fluid may appear on the tip of the penis. Then, liquid from the prostate gland accumulates with sperm from the testicles. At this stage, a man is feeling very sexy but still able to control his response. Finally, the fluid is allowed to enter the urethral bulb through the external bladder sphincter. A delay of a few seconds is followed by the discharge of the fluid in powerful contractions of the Kegel muscles.

PROLONGED ORGASM

As we saw in Chapter Four, one of the big debates in the field of sex is whether orgasm and ejaculation are identical. Obviously, men can ejaculate with little or no pleasurable sensation. But several authors have claimed that men can enjoy a pattern of multiple orgasm just like women. In one sense, this has got to be true. A man can keep making love and experience climax until he has nothing left to ejaculate. He then has what's called a 'dry come' – his body goes through all the motions of attempting to expel fluid, opening the valves and contracting the expulsory muscles but his tanks are simply empty. But, if the external bladder sphincter does not open, this is hard to believe because, if it does open, a man is likely to try to ejaculate.

Perhaps this debate is marginal because when you enjoy your love-life what difference does it make what the labels say? There is certainly a case to be made for prolonging sex by ensuring that men don't come too quickly (unless they are very youthful and therefore able to re-erect quickly and return for second helpings). Whatever men are capable of, women are frequently in the multi-orgasmic league. To ensure harmony with your partner, it's a good idea to find out whether he can manage more than one climax in an hour. (If he can, then it's sensible to see if you can alternate and vary your pleasure sequence).

As men grow older, they commonly complain that climax is less forceful and the pleasurable accompanying sensations appear to diminish. This problem often seems to relate to masturbation rather than intercourse and seems to point up one simple, physical fact – with age men need more sensory and erotic stimulation than a 'routine' episode of personal touch can supply. Excitement is not just a matter of penile rubbing (although the older male will need plenty of that). It's also a question of mood enhancement and knowing your personal, orgasmic pattern. Fantasies may need to be used; time needs to be taken; and if these conditions can be fulfilled a man may find that his orgasm still feels erotically powerful. Of course, the ageing process does affect male

PROLONGING THE MALE ORGASM

There are several tried and tested means of prolonging male orgasm (see also the Squeeze Technique, under Treatments for Premature Ejaculation, in Chapter Four).

- The man should focus on his sensations and stop moving entirely as soon as the pleasure builds up as if to take him over. It doesn't matter how often he does this. It may be a good idea to get him to agree a word to explain what's happening. Partners don't mind when your motive is to increase their pleasure too. Some men simply whisper 'Easy'. Others shout 'Wait!'

- Alternatively, withdraw the penis from the vagina as soon as stimulation becomes dangerously over-exciting. Watch the erection deflate a little then resume the intercourse.

- At the point just before the moment of 'ejaculatory inevitability', go into 'slow motion' mode. Slow all body movements to the minimum.

- Some couples like to 'teeter on the brink' till the man isn't sure whether he's going to come after all. Then the woman flexes her pc or 'Kegel' muscles with exaggerated slowness just tipping him over the edge as her vaginal contractions milk his penis of fluid.

- Other people use sexual leisure drugs like butyl or amyl nitrite, which cause an increase of total blood pressure and serve to prolong and delay the experience of male orgasm. Warning: little pharmacological testing has been done on these products, which are on sale from marital aids shops and via mail-order companies. Doctors expressly state that they should not be tried by those with heart or circulatory disorders. The drug also has to be administered about 30 seconds prior to the desired climax because it is relatively short-acting. Some people also detest the smell of these products.

- Use the 'squeeze' technique or a variant thereof to nip the penile shaft quite hard a couple of times between finger and thumb (or lips) when your partner shows signs of coming. This will delay orgasm while stoking his desire.

- Male orgasm can be delayed or sharpened by having the testicles restrained by hand (holding them away from the body) or by placing a rubber band fixed either at the base of the penis or (gently) wrapped round the base of both penis and scrotum together. Beware of restricting the blood supply or a loss, not increase, of sensation is more probable!

- As we will see in Chapter Eight, the ultimate Male orgasmic hot-spot is the Prostate. This walnut-sized object, accessible via the anus, lies at the base of the bladder and makes a major contribution to all forms of male orgasmic pleasure.

sexual response. But men must understand that before there can be genital pleasure from climax they need to create sufficient muscular *tension* to discharge in their orgasms and this won't necessarily happen simply through casual masturbation at the end of a busy day. Sometimes it takes *your* lips to work wonders.

HOW TO GIVE
GREAT ORAL SEX

As Phillip Hodson has previously written: 'Enjoying oral sex as a giver is about feeling safe and comfortable with what you're doing. There's nothing more natural than taking pleasure in licking, nibbling and kissing your partner's body, even in private places. People have enjoyed oral sex since history began. For instance, the ancient Indian love manual the *Kama Sutra* describes no less than eight different ways lovers can pleasure each other, including one called "sucking a mangoe fruit".'

Hygiene is a foremost concern but the subject can easily become exaggerated. We wouldn't expect you to make love to anyone who was essentially unpalatable and why, therefore, would you make any exception when it comes to kisses below the waist? Washing and bathing can always be included in the preliminaries if you want to be certain of your comfort on this score.

Essentially oral sex needs the performer to be the person in charge so start by getting your partner to make good eye contact then tell him to lie back and relax. The best position for him to be is supine with you seated facing him, your legs stretched out underneath his and *on a bed*. (If you attempt the same sort of lovemaking in a car you must expect to cause undue stress to the muscles and small bones of the neck).

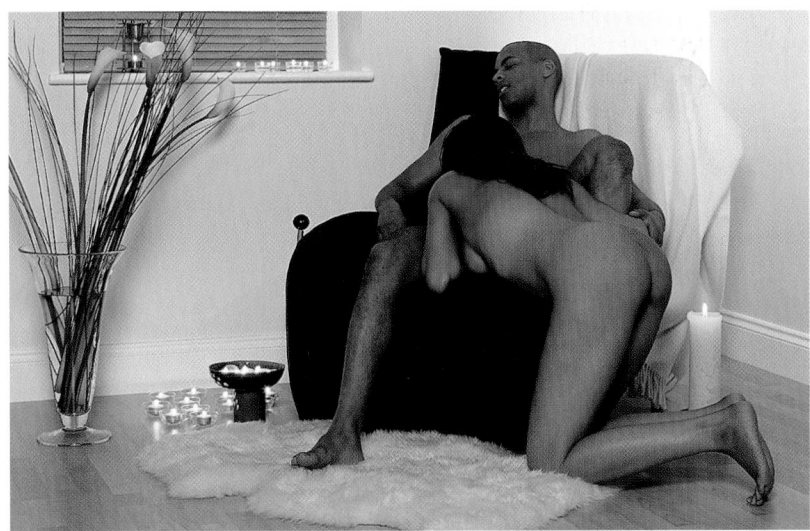

THE FIVE ESSENTIALS IN GIVING YOUR MAN ORAL PLEASURE

1 Be practical and take off your rings and tie back your hair so nothing gets tangled in the action.

2 Don't think of the penis as some sort of fragile orchid. You don't want to scrape any part of it with your bare teeth and do take care when approaching the sensitive penile head and crown. But the rest of the shaft can tolerate hard squeezes and prolonged, vigorous stroking from hands, lips or any other part of your anatomy.

3 Employ your hands to stimulate the penis at the same time as using your lips. This also gives you a buffer on the down stroke.

4 Slide your mouth down over his shaft far enough. Depth of penetration, as the hooker instructress character in Woody Allen's movie *Celebrity* says, is essential. Deep throat is an advanced option – but not everyone is comfortable with taking the penis down towards the wind pipe and breathing only through the nose.

5 You must generate plenty of liquid – lots of saliva – so it's wonderful for him and easier for you.

The best oral sex starts off slowly and deliberately. Only after a while do you speed up. The overall timeframe can be anything from five to fifteen minutes or more. 'What you are aiming to do is build up erotic tension and passion which is then discharged – you're not doing the opposite which is to reduce tension till people lose interest.' For this reason, it is almost always better to go more slowly and lightly than the other person really wants. Eroticism is mostly about teasing and compelling the other person to experience the edge of desire. So we repeat *don't* make a beeline for that genital area at once.

Nibble down from the chest, linger over the skin of the navel, move purposefully across the hips with hot passionate lips, aim for the target then swerve at the last minute towards the inner groin, upper thigh and down to the backs of the knees (by raising your partner's legs) then move up again and make a second pass. Keep the tension high by promising but not delivering till the other person has to *beg* and make sure they don't touch themselves with their hands to spoil the fun.

LOOKING HIM PROVOCATIVELY IN THE EYE...

1 Slowly lower your head and kiss the penile tip. Tease the sides of the shaft with your right-hand fingernails, then form a ring from your fingers and stroke him five or six times.

SAFER SEX

There have been no known cases of HIV transmission through oral sex but herpes can be passed on by kissing of any sort. If you are unsure of your partner's history, a flavoured condom is strongly recommended.

2 Place your left hand firmly around the base of the penis, using loads of saliva over the penile head, and forming your mouth into the letter 'O'. Make sure your teeth are covered by the inside skin of your lips.

3 Slide your lips down the penile shaft till they meet your left thumb and forefinger. Don't rush, prolong his ecstasy. Move slowly and practise sucking with a variety of pressures as you go.

4 As your head comes back up, swirl your tongue across his skin and with your right hand, stroke his balls or inner thighs.

5 To vary the pleasure, place your right-hand thumb and forefinger just below your lips like a second mouth so that hand and mouth move together both stimulating the shaft.

6 Break off from time to time and remind him to 'lose his mind in his fantasies'. He'll know what you mean. Build up erotic tension and increase your speed as his sighs and cries tell you his delight is intensifying.

7 If at the climax, you want to stay with it – fine. If not, keep a box of tissues handy.

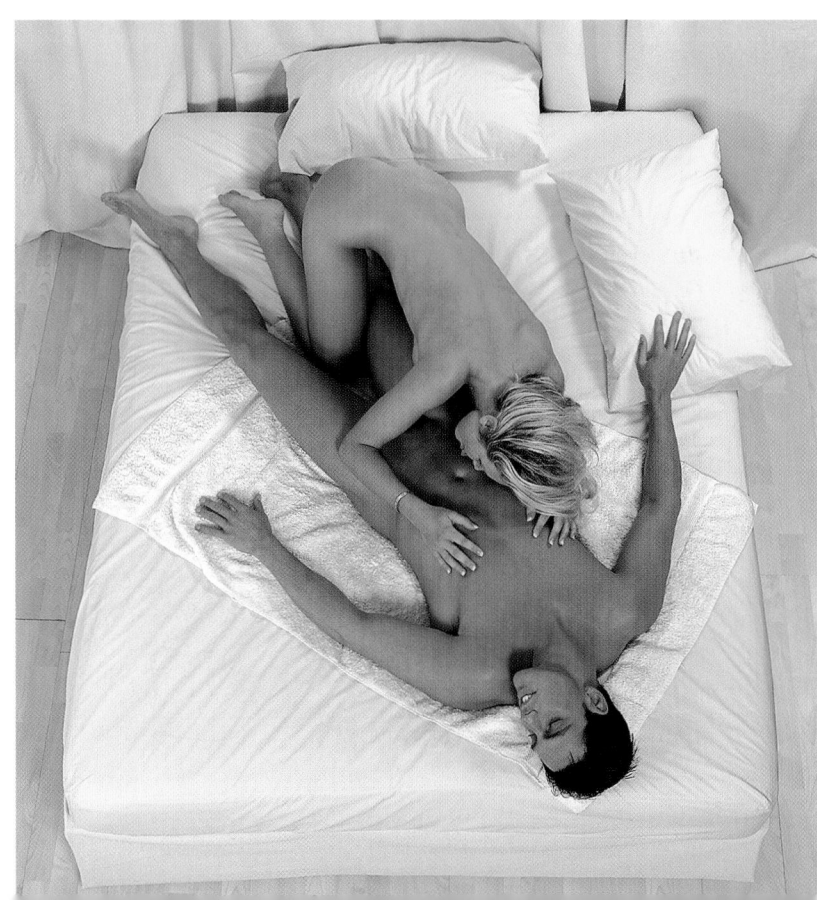

THE BEST ONE NIGHT STAND YOU COULD HAVE WITH A LONG-TERM LOVER

So now you're equipped with loads of news ideas, and lots of straightforward advice, how can you instantly inject your relationship with an emergency dose of passion? Well, no plan, no gain. In any long-term sexual relationship routine will pall. A night of maximum pleasure naturally reverses this trend. But as you'd expect you have to make a little effort. These are the main things you'll need to do.

First, pick your best day – it could be a Sunday. Then make a commitment. Great sex is obviously going to take up a chunk of time and could *even* last for up to five hours. No, don't be shocked. Nobody expects you to perform all-out sex for 300 minutes. But you and your partner need to be sure that there's enough time to make a comfortable transition from everyday concerns and get fully in the mood. Remind him that women are sometimes slower to arouse than men – but once up there, can last a lot longer. So keep patience. And, by agreeing to this sacrifice of time that you would otherwise spend on important activities like watching TV, you both show that you care.

DON'T FORGET THE FOOD OF LOVE
Now, choose the best time of day to do it. A suggestion from experience, would be late afternoon between three o'clock and eight o'clock. Be practical – make sure that you first eat lunch that will sustain you for the labours of love ahead but jointly agree on the menu. Pointers: the food needs to be easy on the stomach and if there's an erotic or romantic significance so much the better. One up-market couple I knew actually had a McDonalds but only because they first met under the sign of the Yellow M. He may want more than a burger, or a crepe suzette.

We stress that it's absolutely vital to protect the time and place from interruptions. Short of installing a force field to block all incoming transmissions, do make sure that the answerphone is on and that Mum cannot phone while you're in the bedroom. Try to make the environment maximise your chances of bliss. This means lighting candles,

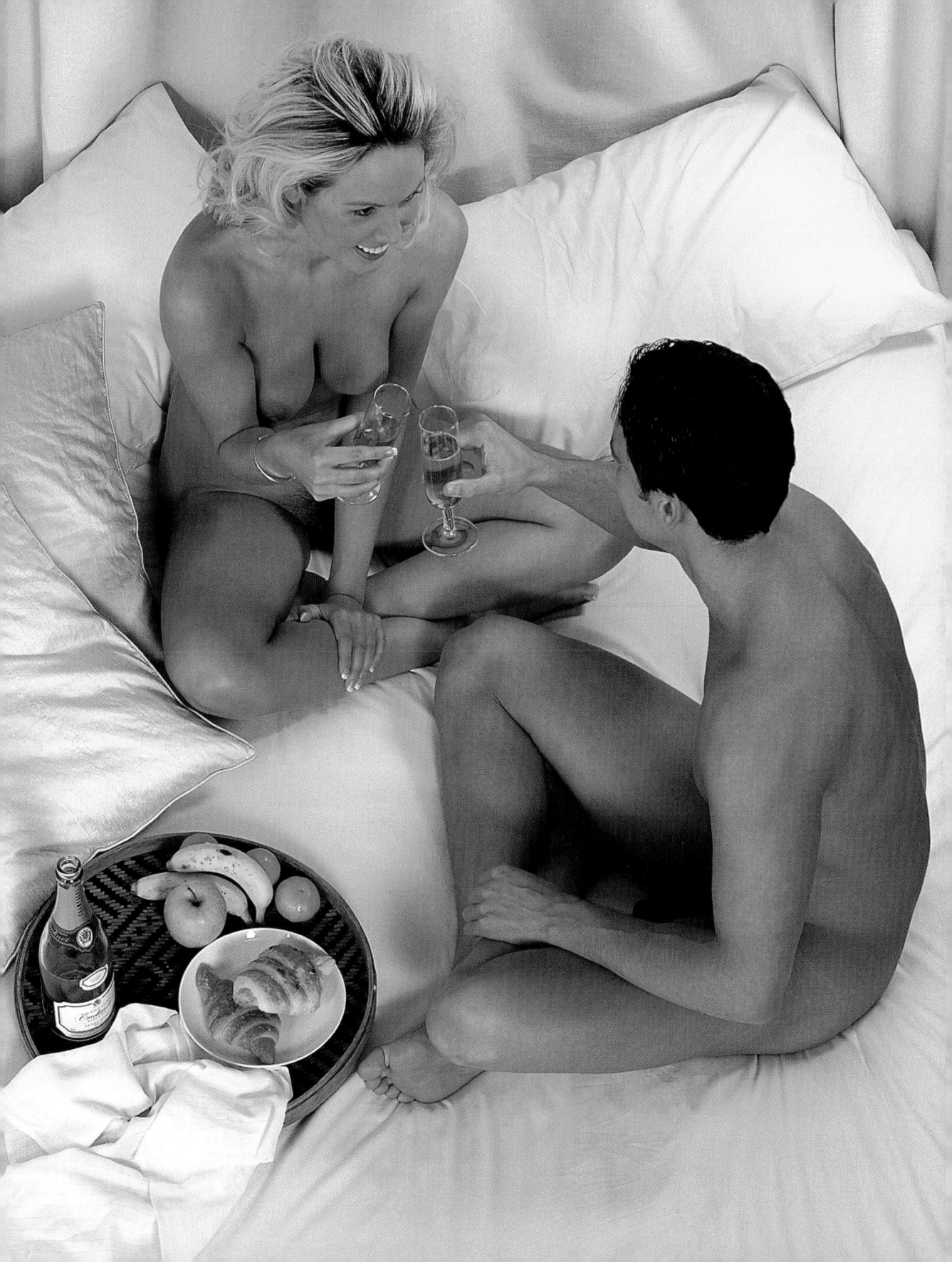

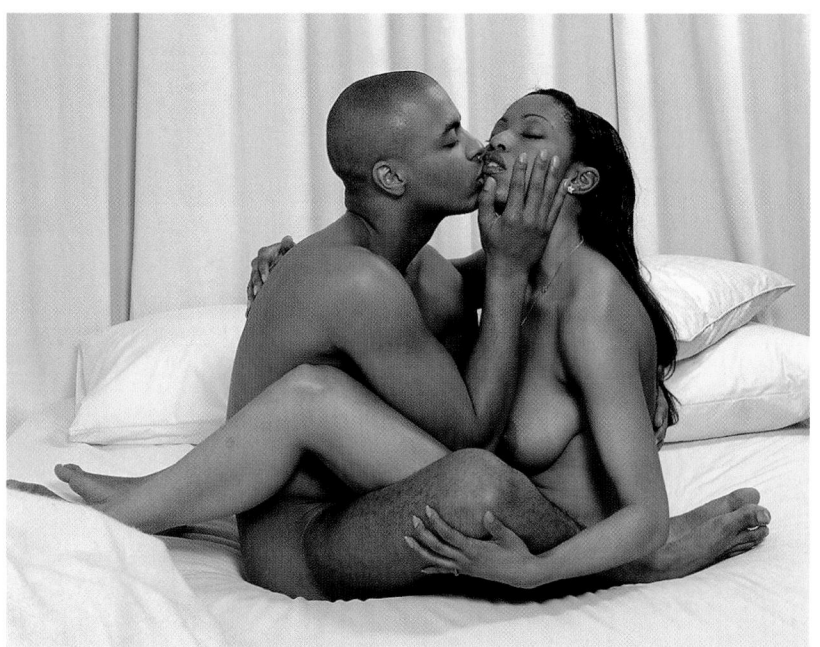

KISSES FOR YOU, TOO

However, avoid being a Victorian lover who makes all the running. Let him kiss you as well, show him how your body likes to be caressed and when he wants to do it guide his hand towards your clitoris to demonstrate the types of touch which give you enough **but not too much** pleasure. It would be a shame to come unless you really want to just yet.

warming the room and playing some old, wistful Sting or Dead Can Dance CDs, or whatever turns you on.

START ... SEDUCTIVELY SLOWLY

Now great sex is slow sex – at least to start with, whatever Hollywood might think. You could begin with a long, lazy shower. Then lead him naked to the duvet in your favourite room – undressing as you kiss – lie down, and let the outside world disappear. Kiss a lot. This is good for him and not bad for you. Stroke constantly. Follow the rules of good massage, and don't let your hands leave your partner's skin. Let the moves flow in a connected sequence. Find those secret non-genital places – like the sides of the neck, arms, legs and chest – and apply a variety of strokes. Don't forget to talk. You can chat while you nuzzle but it's not a bad idea to select subjects related to your feelings about him, how long you've been waiting for this moment, etc. Keep praising him for being able to wait and let the passion accrue.

Now you have to move from stroking the sides of his body while kissing his lips, face and neck to focusing more on the pelvic area. Slowly caress the insides of his thighs, rising higher, with fingers or lips. Or kiss your way from his neck, across the belly, and start gentle oral sex. Don't seek out the penis like the prize in a treasure hunt – 'Gotcha!" Be subtle, kiss or touch the surrounding area first – and a lot. Stroke gently along the edges of the genitals before gradually enfolding the crown with the most featherlight of smooth sliding sucks. You can use your fingers elsewhere on (or in) him at the same time.

STOPPING AND STARTING SEX

Women often ask a silly question: 'How can you tell your partner's ready for intercourse?' The answer is simple: 'When he says "I'll kill you if you don't let me put it in right now".' Quick sex can be wonderful but teasing and frustration are far more arousing. Let yourself be penetrated *slowly*. Build the tension. Use your hand to caress the outside of his buttocks and thighs while he inserts. Try to hold the outstroke for a second till he's had time to realise that you've gone (and time to miss you) then press forward onto him again. Manoeuvre the end of his penis onto the front wall of your G-spot area. Wiggle your hips, pressing harder but ceasing all other movements. Let him reach the edge of orgasm. And slow things down again – still waiting.

Believe it or not, one couple stopped altogether at this point and took a nap. He said – let's see how long we can hold off and she was surprised to be able to relax. But when they woke – she took over, pushed him on his back and rendered him speechless.

The benefit of spending up to five hours on love is that your partner has time to forget all sexual anxiety and inhibition. If you'd like to meet the sensitive soul inside your man, you only need to set the above scene. And we haven't even mentioned humming during oral sex, dusting off the vibrator, tying him up in paper chains he mustn't break, positioning the hall mirror beside the bed, kissing his pheromone-rich armpits, shaving in intimate places, inserting fingers, or using hot towels and cold compresses where the body can safely take it!

THE FURNITURE OF LOVE ...

And during this marathon love-in, we need to re-open a discussion begun in Chapter Two about *where* you are going to make love because it doesn't only have to be in your sleeping quarters.

Think of the many times you've had missionary position sex in bed. All a bit of a blur? Now contrast it with those unforgettable moments of exotic sex that were not in the missionary position and not in your own bedroom – such as in his parents' car, on a Mediterranean beach, in a lift stuck between floors, that little bit of madness at Bangkok Airport.

Think of the first time you were allowed to kiss your long-term partner. Now try to think about the 100th time you kissed him. Or the 1000th. Not quite the same experience is it?

As we have stressed, sexologists and psychologists have proved that sexual quantity and quality decline with repetition. Experiments have shown that where relationships lack sexual novelty the rate of 'mounting activity' dramatically falls. Researchers have called this dependence of libido on novelty the 'Columbus effect' after the man who first discovered the joys of sailing close to the wind at the end of the world.

We can savour two kinds of sexual novelty – with lots of new partners or with new sexual practices and it's frankly easier and safer to concentrate on the latter. Missionary position sex is fine if you want your partner to re-paper the ceiling and work out how many rolls he's going to need. But why is it even healthy to make love in the marital bed at all? The place where you sleep! Where you fall sick! Where you might die!

ARMCHAIR

best position: face-to-face with him seated and you straddling his thighs with your legs hooked over the arms of the chair.

advantages: you start with your legs slightly apart and your buttocks doing wonderful things up his thighs, his hands roaming your back and his lips on your face and breasts. When the pace quickens, make him close his legs, pressurising his genitals while

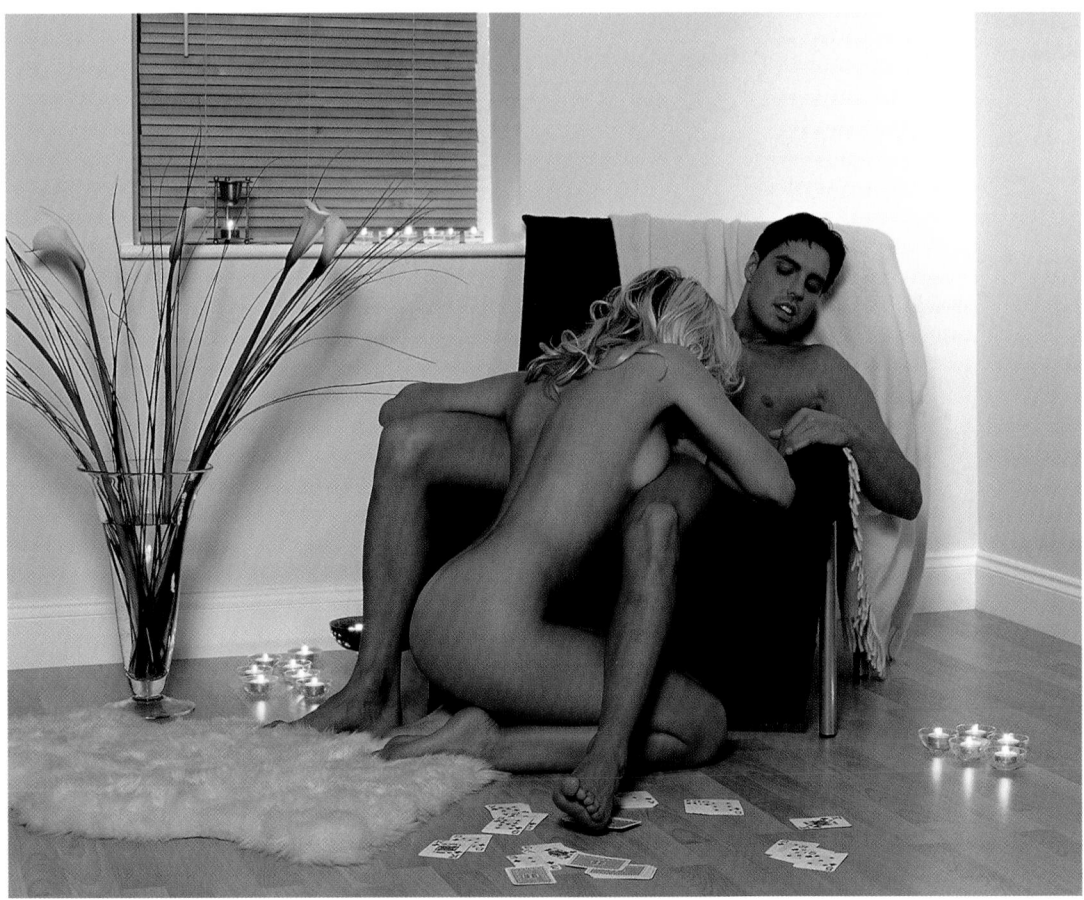

you lower yourself backwards keeping support by holding onto his upper arms. Then slide forwards and backwards along his legs in a comprehensive movement till you can align your G-spot with his glans and the rest is instinct.

precautions: ensure that the seat is sufficiently high to prevent your legs from cramping. If in doubt add extra cushions.

alternative positions that also work:

❣ Rear entry position with one of his legs hooked over the arm of the chair and you seated almost sideways on top of him.

❣ Bent over the arm of the chair doggy-style, him on top, giving instant access to all your sweet spots, your feet perhaps raised to tap erotically on his bum.

❣ Classic oral sex, with one of you seated on the floor, the other swooning in the chair.

BATH

best position: the Thai massage position. For this you'll need masses of mild shampoo or bath foam, a biggish tub, and an initial sense of humour. Fill the bath with five inches of very warm water and make him lie in it. You then pour copious quantities of shampoo etc onto your dry legs, and torso whipping up a lather with the water. You then transfer foam to the front of your belly, lie on top of him, stomach to stomach, and go sweeping up and down his lower abdomen with slightly arched back using your pubic mound as the brush. This can continue until you achieve joint (and jolly hygienic) climax.

advantages: if the massage is carried out properly, geishas in Thailand say no man will remain unmoved.

precautions: it makes sense to avoid drowning. Note: underwater sex is overrated, even for James Bond, though curiosity will doubtless get you to try. If you must do it, be penetrated first then tank up the water level afterwards. Note: water should *never* be forced into the vagina. Avoid tiny, tight tubs.

alternative positions that also work:

❦ Rear entry with woman bending over the side of the tub, dangling.

❦ Spoons with man beneath. Woman gently raises and lowers herself buoyed by the water though careful not to create a tsunami which threatens to empty the bath onto the flat below.

❦ Face-to-face with woman on top, your hands and feet resting on rim of tub. This requires a minimum of 12 inches (of water) and a foam cushion under his bum.

STAIRS

best position: you kneel on the second step from the top of the landing, bottom in the air, body bent forward, head resting on your hands and legs as far apart as stairs permit. He enters your beloved soft spot from behind.

advantages: gives comfortable, all-round support and lots of handholds (other stairs, banisters) for grip and extra thrust.

precautions: never a good idea to lose balance on stairs; also friction or carpet burns can be dicey (though providing trophies).

It's semi-public sex so make sure visiting grannies are not prowling to find the loo after midnight.

alternative positions that also work:

- ❤ You seated with both feet one step lower down, your legs drawn up in the 'birthing' position. You grip both your ankles firmly to add forward thrust to his up-strokes.
- ❤ You sit sideways with your lower leg extended, upper leg bent and top foot inserted between convenient banisters while top hand grasps rail while he gaspingly enters you from behind (vertically or horizontally).
- ❤ You lie on landing facing downstairs your body supported on elbows resting on the second step with legs akimbo – for added pleasure of trying to get your blood to go in two directions at once – to head *and* genitals – and consequent double rush when you finally come.

TABLE

best position: hard to judge because passions and fantasies vary so much. On balance probably best with you teetering on the table edge, legs splayed and underwear removed or pushed aside. He then pleasures you with any of his magic bits – hands, face, whatever.

advantages: since your weight is supported, he enjoys maximal freedom of movement. Also allows for easy and controlled downward thrusts on your clitoris as much as upwards pressure on the anterior vaginal wall for your G-spot. If inclined, he can even describe memorable circles with his buttocks taking you 'round the clock'.

precautions: remove crockery and cutlery. Do not attempt to lie on the table if either party has a bad back. Polished surfaces can be slippery and it is very painful to fall on the floor while locked in coitus – penises in vaginas do break.

alternative positions that also work:

- ❤ Anecdotal evidence says that some men have fantasies about taking their partners from behind 'across the table' eg, while you're preparing a dinner party and already dressed in some finery. Prudence says find out first whether such quickies suit.

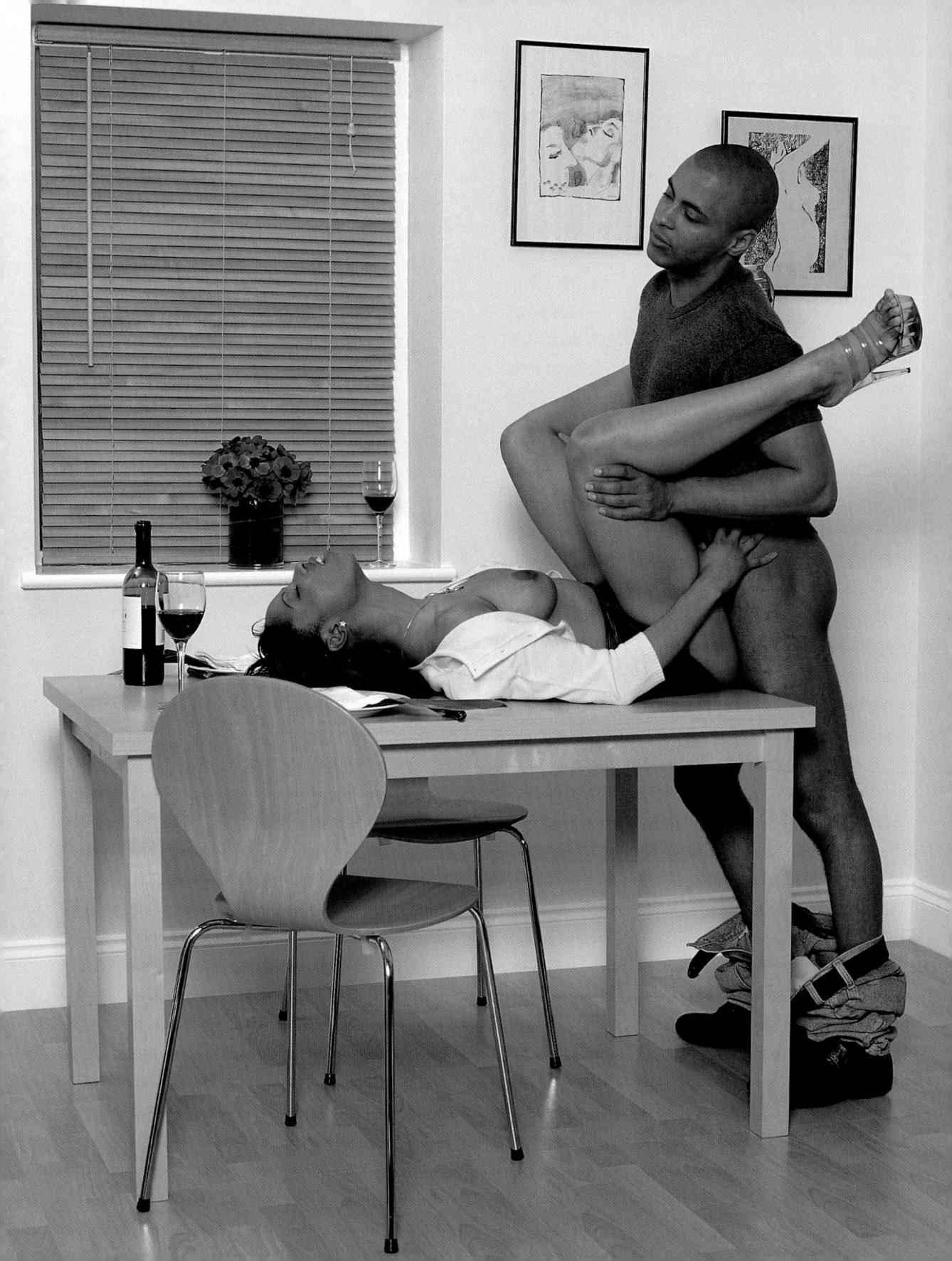

- *Under* the table is a lasting male fantasy. Ideally, you are hidden from view devouring his manhood in the cubby hole of a table that looks suspiciously like a desk at the Oval Office …
- At the restaurant, you slip off one shoe and with your be-stockinged big toe caress his crotch while he eats his soup and goes berserk.

POUFFE/BEANBAG

best position: the moment to try one of those really advanced positions such as 'Hector's Horse' aka 'The Wheelbarrow'. You lie naked with your chest supported by either piece of furniture, your hands flat on the floor while he nimbly inserts himself from behind, grasp your legs and carefully raises your body. Now use your weight to rock forwards and back, building up to a climax of deep thrusts. You also concentrate on exercising your Kegel muscles to milk him of both sperm and sanity.

advantages: visual – his mind is filled with the image of your provocative bottom in a quite pivotal act of penetration. Further allows for double body weight to be brought to bear *genitally*.

precautions: never to be attempted by fourteen-stone feminists on seven-stone weaklings.

alternative positions that also work:
- Squatting. Bean bags offer a sexual platform second to none, moulding brilliantly to your every bodily contour. Here the man places the woman prone or supine across the bag with genitals raised and spread. He then crouches above you, resting his hands on the floor, and attempts to have intercourse without touching you anywhere at all apart from this penetration by penis.
- He sits astride the pouffe while you jockey yourself into position and ride him in the 3.30 at Doncaster – you could let him win by half a length.
- On a bean bag, you lie down with legs raised and thrust back over your head. With your bottom invitingly offered in the air, he penetrates while facing the other way. Holding onto your waist, and rocking gently, the base of his penis and scrotum feather across your clitoris. And so to bed.

8

PERFECT INTERCOURSE... for him

If you want to be literal-minded, of course there's no such thing. But supposing for a moment you could share with your man the best of all possible erotic experiences – and still leave him begging for more – how would the scenes unfold? What would you ultimately do?

Penetration comes in as many different guises as the human body has possibilities. Apart from the obvious, you could explore breasts, buttocks, armpits, feet and thighs. For a man, a sense of completeness lies at the heart of penetrating. Being contained in another body is enclosing, fitting, accepting, embracing, surrounding, joining, merging – as well as opening, achieving, acquiring, manipulating, controlling, effecting – as well as feeling that physically all is aptly in place. The perfect pleasure receptor for a penis is the flesh that enfolds and slides along the penile shaft and head simultaneously. Although men can be boorishly abrupt about foreplay, and insensitively insistent on penetration, you might understand why they place so much emphasis on making an entrance if *your* sexuality also came packaged in an external tube that is looking for its perfect physical receptacle. For the fact remains – *intercourse probably strokes most pleasure receptors in the male brain.*

PUTTING SUGGESTIONS INTO HIS HEAD

To be simple, the primary components of sexual arousal are 'fantasy and friction'. With most men, the fantasy is often triggered, reinforced, overlaid and augmented by the friction. Supposing that on the way to his birthday party in the taxi, you give your boyfriend a wicked look and tell him to stay silent. Meanwhile you unzip his fly and fondle him – for your own pleasure as much as his – and explain why later he will be enjoying the time of his life on your body. But just for now he must put it away. Then you re-zip him as the cab arrives at your destination. He might call you a tease. He might be more than pleased.

This fondling is a totally basic item of foreplay – to tease is to please – but it will also set his mind into a spin of desire. He may even think 'are you someone he has underestimated – do you have more sexual confidence and power than he assumed? Where might this lead?' This process will cause him to have mini-erections (maybe for several hours) and an insistent tug of lust.

THE POWER OF SUGGESTION

You could also take the trouble of assuming he is a connoisseur of sexual visuals. Maybe you have put black underwear on, maybe none. Either way, you have drawn his attention to you – a glimpse of silk or flesh or a visible panty line. Or there may be a question about how well your skirt or trousers hang over your naked buttocks. Something has been suggested to make his mind stay focused on the basics of arousal.

The key to great sex for men lies in the certainty of ultimately gaining an entrance into your body and not being fobbed off with erotic activity that any man can do by himself. Yes, we know this is old-fashioned thinking at one level but to a great extent it remains how men work. Nor does it mean they don't value the remainder of the repertoire. It does *not* suggest they hate game-playing, role-swapping, kissing, cuddling and the whole inventive range of slaps and tickles. But most men most of the time eventually want to press themselves inside your body and come.

So, having aroused him with strokes and carefully selected garments en route to the celebratory feast, you should also let him know he is going to have you tonight, entirely, although there will still be some waiting, some qualifying, some diverting, even some mysterious love-play along the way. But have you he *will* and *may*.

BEWARE

Michael could not believe his luck when he started an affair with Allison. She was good to talk to, friendly, very attractive to him. They got on well both in the gym and in company. At the outset, Allison made all the running. The first thing she ever did was transform an earnest conversation (about her mum) on the couch in her flat into a deep kiss and cuddle. She then crossed one of her legs over his and let her body relax into a sharp, sudden orgasm. Michael found this both totally exciting and exceptionally intimate. She also said she didn't want to sleep with him yet – but was looking forward to being granted the opportunity soon. He was made to wait – and forced to think about it (and her).

The next time Michael saw Allison was at her front door after she had invited him round. She was wearing the total 'Take me to Slut Heaven' outfit – shiny shoes, stockings, short skirt and she flung him down on his back in the hall in her eagerness to mount and come. Unfortunately, she didn't notice that her pace was just a little too much for the more deliberate Michael who was at least ten years her senior. He was being expected to have sexual intercourse a fraction faster than his body could manage. The experience was better for her than him – that vital surrender of self to the moment was missing even though Michael was grateful to feel so enthusiastically appreciated.

There was a worm of worry – could he keep delivering what Allison actually seemed to need? They had their first major disagreement when she picked him up from his office in her car a few days afterwards, late at night, with a view to sex in a nearby lover's lane. Michael, feeling pressurised and somewhat overwhelmed, declined Ally's further advances.

Allison wanted to know what she'd done wrong and in her exasperation muttered the immortal phrase 'So what do men want?' Well, clearly it's not a good idea to assume that your style of sex is exactly what your man is happy with. A little judicious verbal checking is a better policy than that slogan 'All men want is sex and French fries'.

TALKING UP A STORM

Again, this scene is obviously disposed towards the more male view of intercourse but remember that this is his birthday and you still have options (which may make things more personally satisfying). For instance, you might comment: 'I want you to enter me so slowly at first I'm likely to lose control of my mind' or 'I want you to come as fast as you can so I can feel your desire' or 'I want you to hold off from orgasm until I say "Now!".' The approach you choose will depend on what you already know about his sexual psychology – some men are more boosted by easy permission; some by commands; others by a challenge – as well as your own.

PROBLEMS TO AVOID DURING INTERCOURSE

Don't always try to make his thrusting last forever. Men can lose sensation in the penis after 15 or 20 unvaried minutes, which may delay or prevent the male climax. It's wonderful to enjoy slow sex, as we have said, but there needs to be some residual degree of penile friction or a man will find it difficult to sustain his erection. This difficulty also occurs in the woman-on-top position – some men find this position does not provide enough thrusting even to sustain arousal and not everyone is fit enough to thrust from underneath while carrying your weight too.

Find out (preferably beforehand) what your partner likes you to say or not say during intercourse. Some men will relish words of frenzy and desire; some fancy coarse expletives; some like graceful murmurs of approval; some prefer silent appreciation; most love it when you reach climax and signify by some observable announcement that you have actually done so.

We repeat, faking an orgasm is pointless and self-defeating – it's the perfect way to persuade your partner to carry out lovemaking next time that will again prevent you from achieving climax.

At this point, you could place his hand between your thighs for a second then get him to raise the same hand towards his nose to detect the faint but delicious odour of your sexual scent. During the course of the evening, you keep mentioning how excited you feel about what is going to happen when you get home. You could also explain exactly what you have in mind – you want to kiss him at the door, then go upstairs alone to the bedroom, remove your dress, kneel on all fours on the bed and shout for him to come and join you.

ANAL SEX

More nonsense has been talked about sodomy than any other common sexual behaviour. In some American states the term has been legally construed to include unrelated forms of sexual activity, such as cunnilingus. For the record, sodomy means anal intercourse. It has been widely practised by heterosexuals for centuries as a variant or a provocative act of 'deviance' or as a form of contraception. It is also a practice carried out by some homosexuals. If the act is performed with skill it is never painful and often sensuously pleasurable. Both men and women have interconnective nerves and tissue in the region of the perineum and lower pelvis that mean that anal sex can sometimes speedily produce orgasm without any further stimulation. The skilful addition of a little more stimulation by hand to genitals will increase the chances.

Obviously, some people loathe the very idea of this form of penetration because they have developed an acute sense of fastidiousness concerning the by-products of the human condition. But all sex is to some degree about getting wet and sticky and – if anything – vaginal intercourse can be more so.

Psychologically, of course, many males feel an absolute sense of privilege if their experience of intercourse is extended to this traditionally dominant form of penetration. If you are not one of those women who fundamentally finds anal loveplay repellent, and you do not have grounds to suppose that your partner is averse to anal eroticism, then it might be worth your while to begin an exploratory conversation.

OVERCOMING YOUR OWN INHIBITIONS

To repeat: we understand and sympathise with the possibility that you might prefer to give this part of the book a miss. But spare a thought before doing so. Are you 'switching off' because of prejudices that have been sitting inside you since childhood? Do you think, perhaps, that it would be somehow wrong of you to consider this previously dismissed option? Before you make your decision to avoid this activity remember

PRACTICAL SAFEGUARDS

The only practical problems with anal sex are that

❦ care must be taken not to cause physical damage upon entry

❦ safe sex must be practised because the anus can absorb infections and chemicals almost as readily as the mouth

❦ er, that's it.

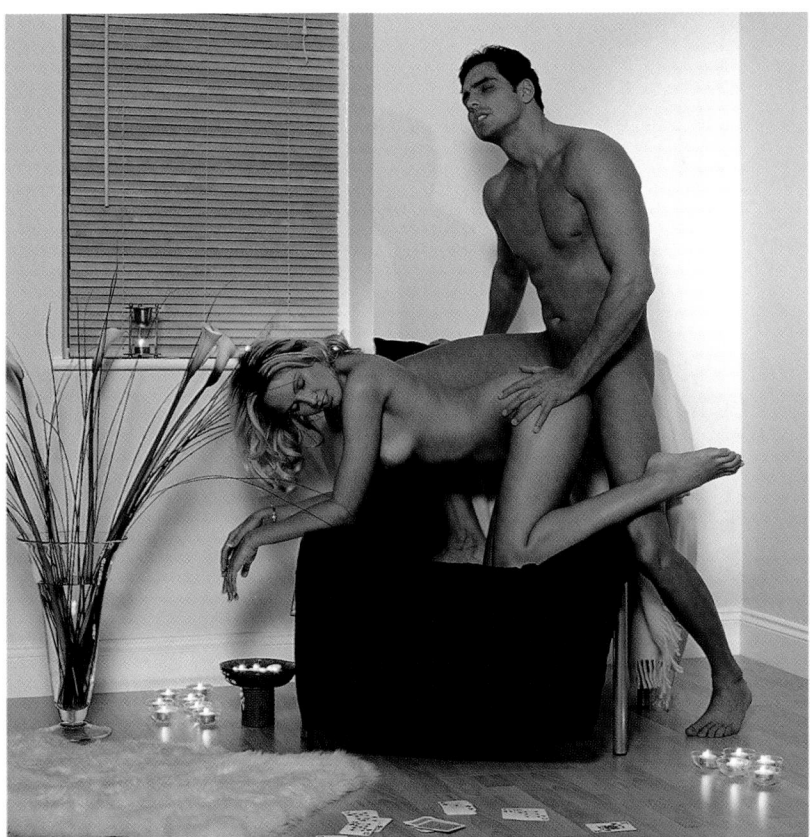

ANAL RULES

- Use an extra-strong condom.

- Use loads of lube – the whole tube if you want. You cannot overdo it.

- Penetrate slowly – he should insert one finger, then two – before attempting to use his penis.

- Let the act be under your total control. You should move onto the man's penis rather than be 'penetrated' by him.

- Ask him to ease back if there is pain. It will stop.

- Pause once penetration has taken place.

- Take as long as you want over this form of sex.

- Re-lubricate if dryness occurs.

- Stop if pain recurs.

- Stop if you get bored!

- Tell him if you love it.

- Ask him to use his hands on your breasts or clitoris as well.

the male aspect. There may be times when you desperately want something erotic done to *you* that *he* may not be keen on. Wouldn't you like him to try and overcome his prejudices for your sake?

Let's be clear. We are *not* advocating that you do anything sexual that you find inherently undesirable. But we are asking that you should do your man the courtesy of continuing to read the rest of this section of the book. We hope it will give you an idea of just how much he might like to explore this boundary (and not only those aspects that are done to you). If you read our later Chapters, you will see that there are some extraordinary strokes you can give to *him*.

HOW TO DO IT

Men, as we have seen, are usually intrigued by 'naughtiness' and rule-breaking so if one day you should purchase some water-soluble lubricant from the pharmacy, and express an interest in pushing the definitions of intercourse in bed, we guess your partner may be compliant or even enthusiastic.

THE MOST PLEASURE YOU COULD EVER GIVE A MAN ...

[One day, the editor of *Cosmopolitan* magazine commissioned an article on men's innermost sexual secrets from Phillip Hodson. The following is the result. She was delighted with the text. Far less happy was the male managing director, who thought no one should read such a 'dangerous' document and withdrew the feature from the magazine at a late stage and great expense. Truth, even inner truth, will out so here you can judge the result for yourself ...].

No woman, not even a doctor, can know how it feels to live inside a male skin. Nor the sort of sexual strokes men really crave. Our friend Steven is a 31-year-old tape and software producer and he's unhappy. For about five years, he's been having an affair with Lise from Frankfurt. They meet as often as money and planes allow. He confesses: 'The relationship's ridiculous. We don't have time for each other. We're not enormously compatible. She wants to talk about West African art. I want to talk about photography and soccer. I feel irritable with her after three or four days of continuous company. But I'm sexually addicted to Lise. In fact, she's spoiled sex for me with anyone else. That woman's so good in bed she's completely ruined my love-life.'

Steven's not the only man to say such things. As you grow up and approach your 30s you run the risk of meeting not only your erotic match but your sexual superior. Lise shares her gift with the earthy character played by Susan Sarandon in the movie White Palace. *Sarandon tells her upmarket boyfriend (snooty James Spader) that 'I may not have a cute little 23-year-old college-educated tush but in the fucking department you ain't gonna find anyone who can blow your brains out like me. On that I'm crystal'. Spader can only reply: 'I've never wanted any woman as much as I want you' and his 'want' has a very big W.*

It's not just in the 'fucking department' that such women appear to have the edge. What happens in the kissing, nibbling, handling and despatching areas is equally vital. Why did Steven fall for Lise? Because on their second date she couldn't keep her hands out of his trousers in the cinema. 'It made me feel simultaneously embarrassed and confident,' he admits. 'On reflection, I loved it.' In White Palace *Susan Sarandon can't wait to go down on James Spader and nothing is going to stop her – not his hangover, not her hangover, not even the perilous shortage of oxygen under the covers. He's edible and she needs him to know.*

Enthusiastic, upfront desire is one requirement. But what really gets a man addicted is when she appreciates how to touch his sexual organs with authority. Of course, there'll be dramas playing aloft – men do bring their brains into bed and there's always a fascinating interplay between the fantasy and friction. However, if you don't start by knowing your genital caresses you'll inevitably ruin the mental sex.

LENGTH AND STRENGTH

It's essentially a question of degree. For instance, when a man has an erection, blood is pumped into the storage reservoirs of the penile shaft, which can therefore sustain high pressure and several hours of pain-free wriggling. In fact, to your surprise, you can grasp the penile shaft and squeeze as firmly as you like without fear of hurting. Bear this in mind the next time he says 'harder and faster' just before coming. A man masturbating will in the final moments apply a fair amount of force and nothing is more frustrating for him at this juncture than manipulation by floppy jelly fingers.

THE MALE CLITORIS

But do not attempt to bend an erection, either at the base or middle when held in your fist. It isn't sexy, it feels like someone is trying to break you in two and you could rupture connective tissue and internal blood vessels. Be equally cautious when it comes to caressing the glans penis, the head of the penis proper, upwards from the coronal ridge. For concentrated nerve-endings, this is the anatomical equivalent of the clitoris. Just as you wouldn't want someone to pretend yours was a sort of Instant Scratch Card, no more does a man want this spot polished until you can see your face in it – especially after orgasm, when any kind of touch to the glans is *intolerable*.

Beneath the glans, there's a ligature called the frenum or frenulum, a sort of rubber band of flesh joining the glans to the undershaft. This responds to the kind of caresses that you might like applied to a nipple. What I mean is that while ecstasy may be achieved, sensory overload is also a risk. Touch by fingers, tongue, nose or toes should be lightly measured, conservative rather than radical. Biting is a very bad move. As a matter of information, Roman mistresses applied dried nettles at this point to cause the man a constant itch of desire, thus stinging their partners into added frenzy. (Use young green nettles *only* if you've explored alternative means of ending your relationship, and don't mind being sued).

THE INTERNAL G-SPOT

The ultimate (internal) Male G-Spot is the Prostate. (if you can distinguish a sex position from a love-juice gland you won't pronounce this 'prost<u>R</u>ate'.) This walnut-sized object, accessible via the anus, lies at the

THE INTERNAL APPROACH

It's the internal approach to a man's G-Spot that provides most opportunities to spoil his love-life forever with anyone else – as Dr K. R. Stubbs describes in his book *Romantic Interludes – A Sensuous Lover's Guide* (Secret Garden Books, California, 1986):

1 'When his feelings become more intense, concentrate your right-hand movements on the area just below the pubic bone and above the anal opening. Using the flat of your fingers in a paddle-like shape, put a firm pressure on this cavity. Now make small circles so that his skin moves over the muscles beneath.

2 'Next make very delicate circles with a finger tip around the anal orifice. If you are finding it difficult to reach, you can ask your lover to bring his right knee upward so you can brace it with your chest.

3 'Whenever he becomes really turned on, your longest finger (with a smooth short fingernail) begins to enter the anal opening. Until the sphincter muscles become accustomed to this touch, your lover may find the sensations intense.

4 'So rather than sliding the finger directly in,' says Dr Stubbs, 'begin a gentle rocking motion. Giving small gradual stretches, you invite the muscles to relax. Remember to use plenty of oil.

5 'When your finger is in full length, try a 'come here' stroking with the finger pad against the tissues on the upper area at twelve o'clock. Here is the approximate position of the prostate gland. Depending on the length of your finger, you may feel a firmer spongy tissue a little different from those surrounding it.'

'If his groans sound deeply happy, don't worry about the exact anatomy ...' because you've reached his goal. The man is yours.

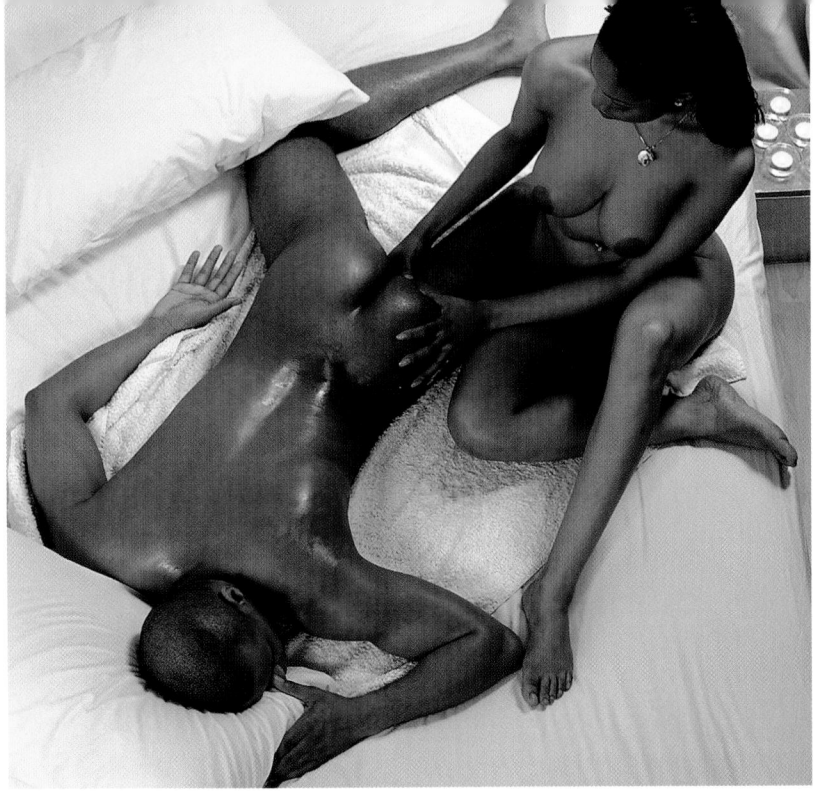

base of the bladder and contributes additional secretions to the seminal fluid. For instance, when a man is erotically teased but prevented from climaxing, there may appear at the tip of his penis a tiny pearl of colourless prostatic liquid.

The prostate mysteriously enlarges with age and is prone to cancer although the 'PSA test – prostate specific antigen' (cost, negligible) can detect both difficulties, in case he wanted to know. Palpation by proctologists is a traditional method of checking for abnormalities and can result in functional orgasm without erection. Palpation by a lover (wearing a surgical glove) is a guaranteed method of sending a mortal male to heaven and can be broached either externally or internally.

APPROACHING THE MALE G-SPOT FROM THE OUTSIDE

To stimulate the prostate from the outside, trace the contours of that narrow divide called the perineal gap between testes and anus. This tissue also contains the pelvic floor muscles which contract during climax. Firm digital pressure (rigid middle finger supported by adjacent fingers) rubbing at the central midpoint of this gap can help arouse a man and remind him of the forthcoming delights of orgasm. He's unlikely to climax but he can certainly go a long way towards it.

WAYS TO USE YOUR NEW SKILLS

If your partner has been especially deserving, then the following reward may be granted:

- ❦ After warm and wonderful sex (during which you alone are permitted to reach orgasm), the man (now a little tired) is asked to lie on his back.
- ❦ You adopt a seated position facing him, your legs extended under his – his thighs wide-spread and loosely wrapped around your waist. His erection should be manipulated by finger tips, fist and lips.
- ❦ Large amounts of appropriate oil or water-based lubricant permit one finger to find the prostate gland as in Dr Stubbs' description.
- ❦ Then the movement of the internal finger is co-ordinated with the gentle rocking motions of your head or hands over the penile head and down the shaft as your choice or his wild whimperings may indicate. You are now in sole charge of both male G-Spots, the underside of the penile head and the deep-rooted prostate. Try to catch the exact and precise *slow* syncopated rhythm that will make him putty in your paws.

If there is any information about his life or past lovers you feel he has ever withheld from you, this is an excellent time to find answers. The male ejaculatory reflex consists of two pleasurably co-ordinated phases. In the first, the prostate suddenly hardens. Your lover approaches his point of no return. (You could of course, cease moving altogether if still seeking confessions). The autonomic nervous system gathers fluid from the prostate and testicular tubes, adds sperm from the seminal vesicles and in one delicious spasm passes all to a collecting node at the base of the penis. The process is called emission. Your man is now going to come and there is nothing you can do about it – threatening him with death won't change a damn thing. Your one choice is to decide in the next five tenths of a second how you want to arrange your body as he finales. Oh yes, he'll howl. Later he'll say 'You got me'. But that's what you probably wanted to hear.

This is where that (in)famous *Cosmo* article ends. We find it interesting that the *female* editor wanted to include it while the *male* proprietor did not. We honestly feel we are informing women about something they would like to know – even if their choice of action may ultimately be *not* to do it. The choice is up to you and lies in your own hands.

HIS 14 ALL-TIME FAVOURITE EROTIC TREATS

1   Provoke a quickie – you stay fully clothed (though thoughtfully without panties). He strips naked.

2   Or leave your panties on during sex so he has to push them aside. The extra stimulation on the side of his penis from the elastic can be thrilling but not from your tightest pair.

3   See if you can make him hard without touching his penis at all (or him touching or pressing against you). Keep mouthing the words 'I want you inside me, please' but don't let him near you. Remember, verbal stimulation only.

4   Slip him inside then command 'Don't move'. Stop him thrusting but allow the occasional 'sway' or 'rocking' motion so he can remain erect. Make him close his eyes with you and slowly synchronise your breathing till you can last 45 minutes. Then, go berserk.

5   When you remove your bra, take his head in your hands till his ear is placed right over your heartbeat and he can listen to your desire.

6   During mutual masturbation, practise treatments for premature ejaculation on your lover for fun. Keep this interesting hand-job going for half an hour – with or without oil.

7   Gently pinch his nipples then ask him if he'd like you to do it 'harder or softer'. There could be surprising answers.

8   Manipulate his testicles and see if they will both fit into your mouth at the same time or just one at a time, then suck gently. Find out if he also likes to be (gently) squeezed.

9   Ask him to kiss you all over while you use your vibrator to come.

10   Then use your vibrator to make him come – applying the point to the underside of the head of his penis and kiss him.

11   Handcuff your partner then use eyelashes and tongue to tease his skin all over. Tell him he can only have firmer touches if he says the words 'I surrender'.

12   Put lipstick round the end of his penis then suck it off.

13   Wear a free-flowing skirt and no panties. Give him a face massage while sitting astride on his chest, with your skirt over his head. Keep moving your body forward so he has to inhale your perfume. Create the impression you might sit on his face.

14   Dim the lights so he cannot see your face, strip off and sit on a chair. Tell him if he stays on the other side of the room he can watch you reach climax.

KEEPING INTERCOURSE SCRUMPTIOUS

Although keeping things exciting and sensual is as much about conversation as fornication, playing games in bed has its place. There actually are times when the way to a man's heart is via his penis. Provided you are both eager to enhance what you've already got, it's always worth thinking up new angles on what goes in the bedroom.

BEDROOM DESIGN

We are often curiously unadventurous when it comes to bedroom design. Considering that bedrooms are also sex rooms we tend to keep them curiously asexual. It could be time to change this.

- ❦ Declare that you are going to 'dowse' the bedroom for genuine ley lines. This involves picking up a pair of cheap dowsing rods at your nearest 'new age' shop. Seeing them in action is quite startling. They certainly give the impression that they work. (And even if they don't, the point here is that you are putting new ideas into his head.) As you walk slowly across the room with the dowsing rod outstretched it appears to be possible to pick up certain surges of energy. What's more, once you've found the energy it also seems to exist in lines. When you identify these lines stretching across the room, move the bed so that it is emphatically *not* in the path of one of the lines. The sexual implication is that you are likely to enjoy much more sensual and relaxed love-making as a result. It's a kind of Celtic 'feng-shui'.
- ❦ Moving the bed anyway makes an interesting and subtle difference. Something about seeing the floor or the ceiling from a new angle.
- ❦ Too much domesticity damages novelty. Changing the colour of the light bulb in the bedroom can cast a new light on the proceedings. So too can the use of candles on an occasional basis. Invest in clusters of these, which you place at key points of the room so that their flicker casts areas of light and shadow.
- ❦ If you can afford to do so, consider changing the bed. Most of us stick with the same old thing for year after year. But styles in beds change too. One of the most interesting designs to hit the market recently are the gothic iron variety. Invest in a gothic four-poster

and yards of red muslin material. This latter you can drape and wind around the posts and overhead frame so that with a background of shadows there is a distinctly Translyvanian tinge to the proceedings. Make sure the mattress is hard enough for sex; intercourse needs grip so your knees and elbows are stable. Some lovers also consider applying eye hooks to the bedframe to fit ropes and scarves etc.

- Is the bedroom décor too girly? Think of a bolder colour scheme – reds, greens, blacks, something that would fit in with the Count Dracula look.
- Get a VCR for the TV so that you can watch something intimate. Put a bolt on the door to keep the world and family at bay. Buy warm, curly rugs. Get slinky, shiny sheets. Supply suggestive sexual accessories – oils, essences, perfumes, flavoured creams, sex toys. Make sure that the room can be heated since cold sex is not just unpleasant but sometimes impossible.
- If you hate the idea of doing this to the room that you sleep in, consider converting the spare room instead. The notion of having a sex room is erotic in itself – call it anything from a playroom to a dungeon!

BUILDING UP TO SEX

- Breathing sweet nothings into your lover's ear while he is at work can make him desperate to get home at the end of the day. Sometimes it's easier to be sexy when you can't touch your lover or see him face to face, so get dialling – 'Hello, would you like to hear what I've just done? I've taken all my clothes off and I'm lying on the bed with my legs held tight together waiting for you to come home and prize them apart' would be simple but satisfactory …
- Tell your lover, at least once a day, what you love about him. And make sure this regularly includes something very personal and private. Even if it's difficult to voice, make the effort. 'It's the way your jeans strain across your manly figure … ' or 'It's remembering how hard your thighs feel' or 'I love your cock when it rises to me.'
- Tell him one of your sexual fantasies in return for one of his. For example: I have accompanied you to a group sex party. I'm terribly nervous because I've never been to one of these before and

you have promised to be very gentle towards me. But I know that you nevertheless intend to get into a threesome with me and even as I look around the room I see you beckoning to a really beautiful red-headed woman who is wearing nothing but a velvet ribbon around her neck … '

🐛 Telephone your partner and pretending to be someone else, arrange to meet him for a first date in a pub. When you arrive for the drink, ensure that you are dressed 'in character'. Perhaps you are playing a working-class hooker and have put on fishnet tights and shiny heels. Or a glamorous society type where you are wearing evening dress. He might be the captain of a ship in smart naval blazer with brass buttons or a working-class gigolo in stripy tee-shirt and French beret.

🐛 If you've got the cash, sharpen up your wardrobe and invest in gorgeous underwear. Men love women in silk – silk slacks with silk underwear underneath makes for pure seduction. Stand with your back to him so that he can see the outline of your no-pantied buttocks against the silk and tempt him towards touching. Surprise him in bed by keeping your clothes on instead of taking them off. Practically anything that's black, lacy and figure-hugging will do. If you want to play the bride, invest in white lacy knicks and lace-topped self-grip stockings. But underwear needs to be *seen*. So don't always sit – how to put this – in a ladylike manner. Remember Liz Hurley's dress that was split up the front so high a deliberate glimpse of sequinned panties was shown. Liz is a potential role model.

GOING TO BED

🐛 The right time for sex is when you *feel* like it. If sex has always been part of a bedtime routine, inveigle him into your arms during the hours of daylight. If you meet with resistance to this idea, either from him or from *you*, do it anyway. The whole point about re-vitalising a sex life is to experience newness. And having sex when you are not even sure you want it because you haven't prepared for it in the usual way, is a new feeling. Just explain you urgently need him inside you so could he lie down, please, while you enjoy an orgasm?

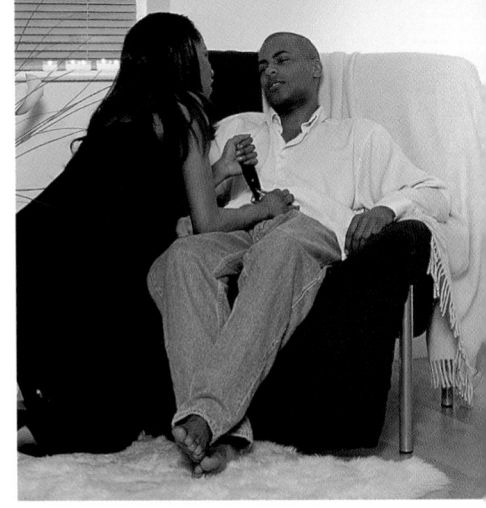

❦ Go to bed *before* you get tired. If you only ever make love when you are exhausted it's hardly surprising it doesn't work very well. If you habitually get ready for bed on a kind of auto-pilot, deliberately do it differently. Run him a bath and share it with him. Shower together. Fool around with the spray nozzle and shampoo. The *Kama Sutra* includes shampooing as one of the high erotic arts (before the days of indoor plumbing). It's a practice we appear to have forgotten. So get in there with the foam. Give your partner the kind of sensitive soaping he's only had in his dreams.

❦ Make love in the living-room. There's a hint of risk and exposure – bodies sliding off the sofa onto the living room rug, clothes pushed aside, hands grasping hips, mouths hungry for kisses, hair in a tangled mess … and are the curtains completely closed? There isn't any chance someone will come in through the door, is there? Or is there?

CHANGING THE ROUTINE

❦ If he has always been the sex initiator, take gentle charge yourself. Lead him in to your newly darkened bedroom and softly, sensuously, undress him. Unbutton his shirt, unzip his trousers. Don't let him do anything for himself. If he objects, point out that this is an experiment with a new approach. Tell him gently but firmly that to be a truly sensual being you need to learn to accept sex as well as give it. Surely he wants to be a well-rounded sexual personality, doesn't he? If he argues, take it in turns to be in charge.

❦ Make a point of approaching sex in a way that is clearly different to the usual routine. For example, if you have paid little attention to stimulating parts of his body other than his genitals, do so now. On the other hand, if you have avoided giving his penis a digital massage, now is the time. Best of all of course is to do both. Aim to stimulate your partner so much that he is desperate for you to go further. But be aware that going further does not have to mean having intercourse. For a change, going further might mean carrying on with the hand stimulation until it reaches the ultimate conclusion. Don't get annoyed because this leaves your satisfaction out of the proceedings. Tell yourself that it is often good to focus exclusively on your lover's experience and that your turn will come. At a later date you can ask him to return the compliment, offering you an evening where love-making is for your pleasure alone.

❦ Some people discover they are immensely turned on by the thought of vicarious pleasure, the idea of seeing another couple making love. The trouble is, this isn't so easy (or safe) to arrange; indeed perhaps you know that the reality is just not an option. The next best thing can be catching a glimpse of the two of you in the mirror. It can be surprisingly like watching another couple. Here's a blue movie for your eyes alone. Setting up a large mirror next to the bed or at the end of the bed can be passionately erotic.

❦ Tape record the sounds of lovemaking and play them back the next time you go to bed. Of course you must both agree to this or it's a non-starter. Some people are specially turned on by sounds. Eavesdropping on your own groans of pleasure and desire can start you off with a rush.

❦ Word of warning: although many couples love the idea of video taping themselves in bed, it isn't clever. Once a sex film exists, in which you can be clearly identified, there is always the potential for unpleasant exploitation. Men and women really have been horrified to discover their home movies circulating down at the bar or club where everyone knows them. Or even on television. Resist the temptation.

❦ Fur, feathers, latex, satin, tantalise your lover's skin with textiles. One of the most original ideas we heard of was the shaving brush sex aid. Take an old-fashioned shaving brush, cut a circle of bristles from the centre, and brush your man's nipples or penis with it, again and again. And there's still latex, satin, feathers, fur and silk for next weekend time.

❦ As we've said, chart the unknown territories of your lover's body. Just because you've been sharing life and love for years does not mean you know every single part of their body as intimately as you think. Couples are often astounded by the new information they find out about each other by playing the game of Find the Erogenous Zones. The secret is to touch every single part of their skin, even the areas that you think cannot possibly be sexy. Ask 'Do you like that? Did I score?' And get your partner to rate your touch on a plus or minus scale. Good touch rates up to Plus Three. Little reaction is zero. And poor or uneasy reaction rates as Minus Three. You can, using this method, build up a kind of relief map of each other's hot spots across the body.

- Play at acting out a script. There's the 'I'm the glamorous career woman who is interviewing you, a beautiful young man who is so desperate for a job that he will agree to do *anything*, however unusual it might be. This might include slowly stripping in front of me. You are completely mine to command.'

- Play the Sexual Picnic game. The living room is your grassy meadow and in your hamper is a feast of exotic fruits beautifully laid out on small silver salvers. After you have fed him exotic titbits and offered him champagne, you lead him to the stream (the nearest warm and ready-prepared bath) and taking his clothes off, you let him soak. Pour more champagne into his mouth followed by strawberries covered in ice from the fridge. After cradling him in the bath and slowly soaping him, you slowly strip off. Offer him warm fluffy towels and after drying him take him back to the meadow. On a large picnic blanket (a towel) lay yourself out. You are the table and on your body is placed an array of succulent substances. His task is to eat them from off your body without using his hands … You get the idea.

- Rent a sex video and set up the video player and screen so that you can watch from bed.

- Agree to listen to any (repeat any) sensual request your partner makes tonight, without laughing, criticising or flinching. You don't have to do it, but if you consent, it might revolutionise your relationship: 'For years, I've wanted you to … slowly at full stretch … and wear nothing else in bed … '

Sometimes of course people wish to move from a simple scene into more elaborate and explicitly choreographed games. The next chapter gives you a few script ideas for your own roleplays.

9

GAMES AND Scenes TO MAKE GROWN MEN WEEP

It stands to reason that if you want to experience great physical sex you need to receive some great mental sex. What gets dissipated at orgasm is tension from both body and mind. Therefore, the more obstacles you can place in the path of instant gratification, the more pleasures you can ultimately enjoy.

Physical caresses that go on for ages with subtle, prolonged permutations help prepare you. So do those tormenting thoughts of 'so near and yet so far'. The art of love is the art of timing. This chapter shows you how to improve this timing by using the dynamics of restraint to bring your partner close to ecstasy. Of course, too much frustration will generate a kind of disappointed boredom. But if you follow these detailed guidelines you'll get your timing absolutely hot spot on.

THE RULES

Before you start

1   Do not play these sorts of games with anyone you distrust or have only just met. The purpose of the activity is to extend the boundaries of an already close relationship. You are using your private knowledge of your partner to get further into their mind as well as body, so there is no point in even contemplating a casual encounter.

2   Both parties must be willing. It is out of the question to suggest these games to someone who has claustrophobia or suffers nightmares about sexual control.

3   Before the first knot is tied, agree an emergency phrase or code to be used if either person wishes to bale out. Sometimes, this will not be a word but a gesture or a specific cry.

4   Do not attempt these games with those who are in poor health.

5   Do not restrict airways or use restraints that prevent the proper circulation of the blood.

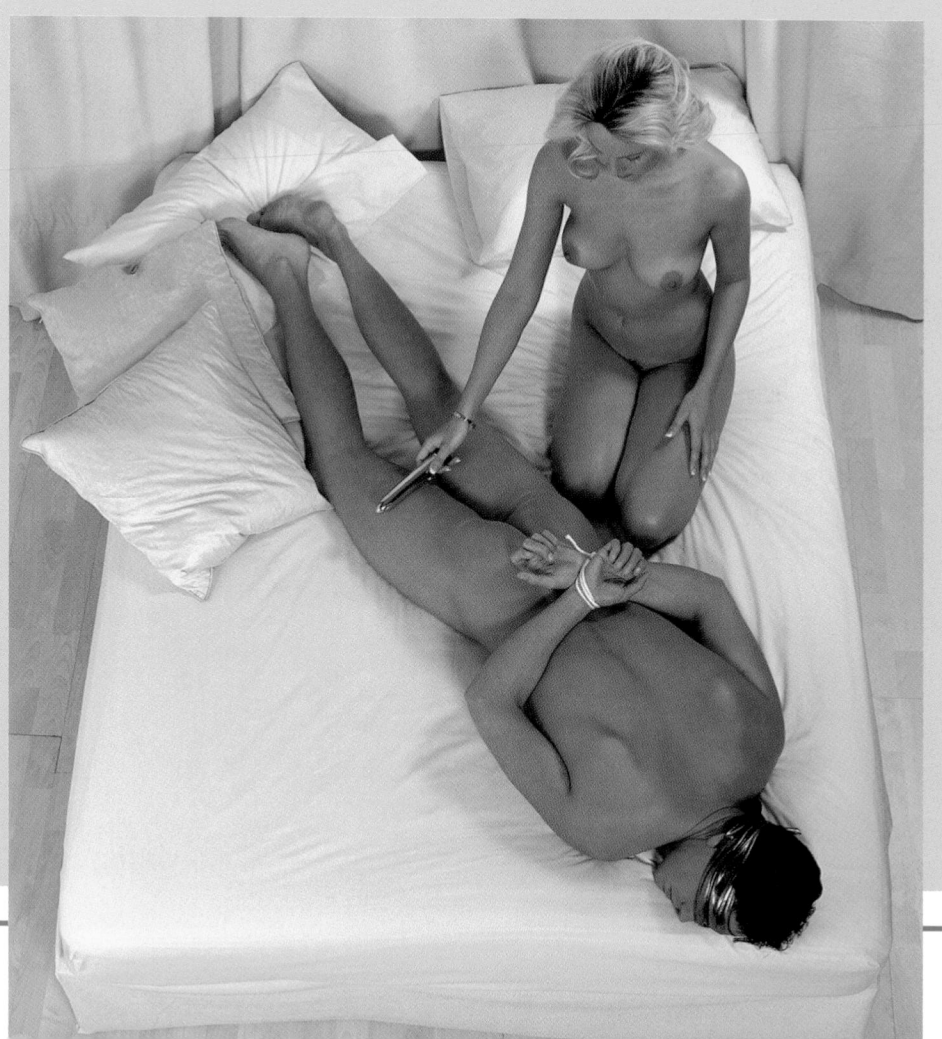

Research suggests that powerful, successful people of either sex are those likely to enjoy some form of part-time psychological surrender.

CREATING THE RIGHT MOOD

Every relationship has a 'balance of power'. Different people have different skills and areas of knowledge. Perhaps a woman can speak more authoritatively on matters of tax law and a man on contraception – or it could be the other way round. Different people also have different levels of energy and desire. On some occasions you may feel like urgently initiating sex; on others you may want to be pampered and let your lover take the strain. We all had a special relationship with the first authority figures in our lives, our parents. And the memories they gave us from childhood can colour our deepest sexual wishes and fantasies.

So when thinking about broaching the subject of gentle erotic bondage, ask yourself about this balance of power in your partnership.

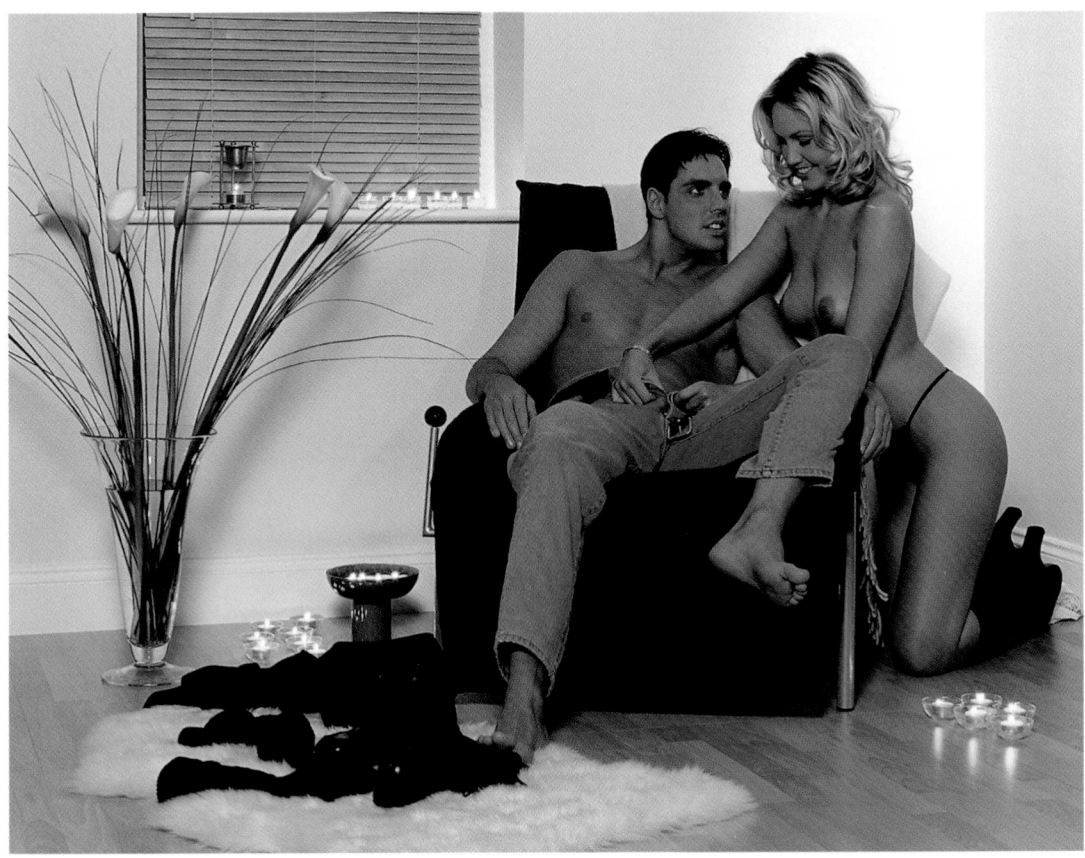

PROPS YOU MAY NEED

🍓 Be subtle. In the coming weeks, you can lead up to the use of more formal items but the first time, keep everything ultra simple. A beautiful chiffon scarf can be used to bind hands. Perhaps you will want more than one. Maybe you can wear stockings which, once removed, can be pressed into service as ropes?

🍓 If you want to bind your partner to the bed, think about where the ties will be tethered. Practise in advance to be sure they will hold. You can secure useful hooks into the underside of a bed-frame.

🍓 Buy a sleep blindfold. Perhaps start using this routinely when you go to bed 'to curb glare'. This will then be handy on the bedside table when you want to initiate a game.

🍓 As mentioned in Chapter 6, massage gloves faced on one side with velvet and the other with fake fur can be obtained and are a wonderful secret weapon to use on your partner's flesh as he/she lies naked, restrained and blindfolded before you.

🍓 Other useful accessories include earplugs, or headphones from a Walkman (if you want to close another of your partner's senses), warm oil and (possibly) ice cubes.

Has the other person ever shown the slightest tinge of interest in erotic control or surrender? Does your instinct tell you to proceed with ultimate caution or could you be pushing at an already half-open door? Clues would include your joint physical behaviour. Have you ever indulged in mild wrestling games together or enjoyed occasional slaps and pats on the bottom as you pass from one room to the next? Is your partner happy to accept forceful touchings and teasing even when sex isn't on the menu? When in bed, does he relish the thrill of prolonged foreplay or generally precipitate to speedy orgasm? Is he the sort of person who has ever hinted at a desire 'to feel submissive'? Is he the sort of guy who has ever shown the faintest desire to fall at the feet of 'domineering women'?

All these are the sorts of potential openings to explore if you intend to seize the moment. Nothing ventured, nothing gained. The type of gambit you might try is 'Funny you should say that. I'd love to take total charge of you tonight. I want to make you weep with pleasure. There's only one difficulty in the way. Will you let me?'

MOVES YOU TWO MIGHT MAKE

These are the suggested moves and scripts you might follow on a first attempt to introduce more mood heat into your bedroom. The tone should be gentle and trusting and the voice kept low and seductive till the receiver is 'secured'.

gaining permission: It's a good idea to begin making love to your partner in the usual way. Ensure he is highly aroused, warm, sexy and full of desire.

furthering your suggestion: Build a picture in words of how you enjoy touching and stroking his most secret recesses but don't exactly match words to actions. Stroke *near* but not *on* the places he most wants you to touch. The key to success is 'frustration of expectation'. Get him used to you not touching his most sensitive zones then accidentally let one finger wander and trail ever so lightly across the genitals. If you're doing it properly, he should gasp.

raising the temperature: Now you want to suggest to your partner that it's time for a little extra surrender: 'Would you like to feel unlimited pleasure, to go almost crazy with desire, to feel helpless with passion? You would? Then keep your hands over your head while I get to work.'

the takeover: However, it's very difficult to keep your hands constantly above your head while being frustratingly teased just off centre below the waist so eventually your victim is likely to disobey. Now you suggest a solution. 'Will you do as I ask? Will you put your wrists together and let me tie them so I can really give your skin bliss and make you entirely happy without all these tedious interruptions which neither of us want? Please? Will you do that for me?' (Hands can also be tied to the bed/bedframe/headboard for complete security – and feet likewise if you both see fit. On a first occasion, remember 'less may be more!' And you also want to have something to look forward to).

knots reprise: Use the scout's reef knot – 'left over right and through; right over left and through' because you can always undo this easily by pulling open one of the loose ends and slipping off the remaining loops. (Finally Girl Scout training has its uses...)

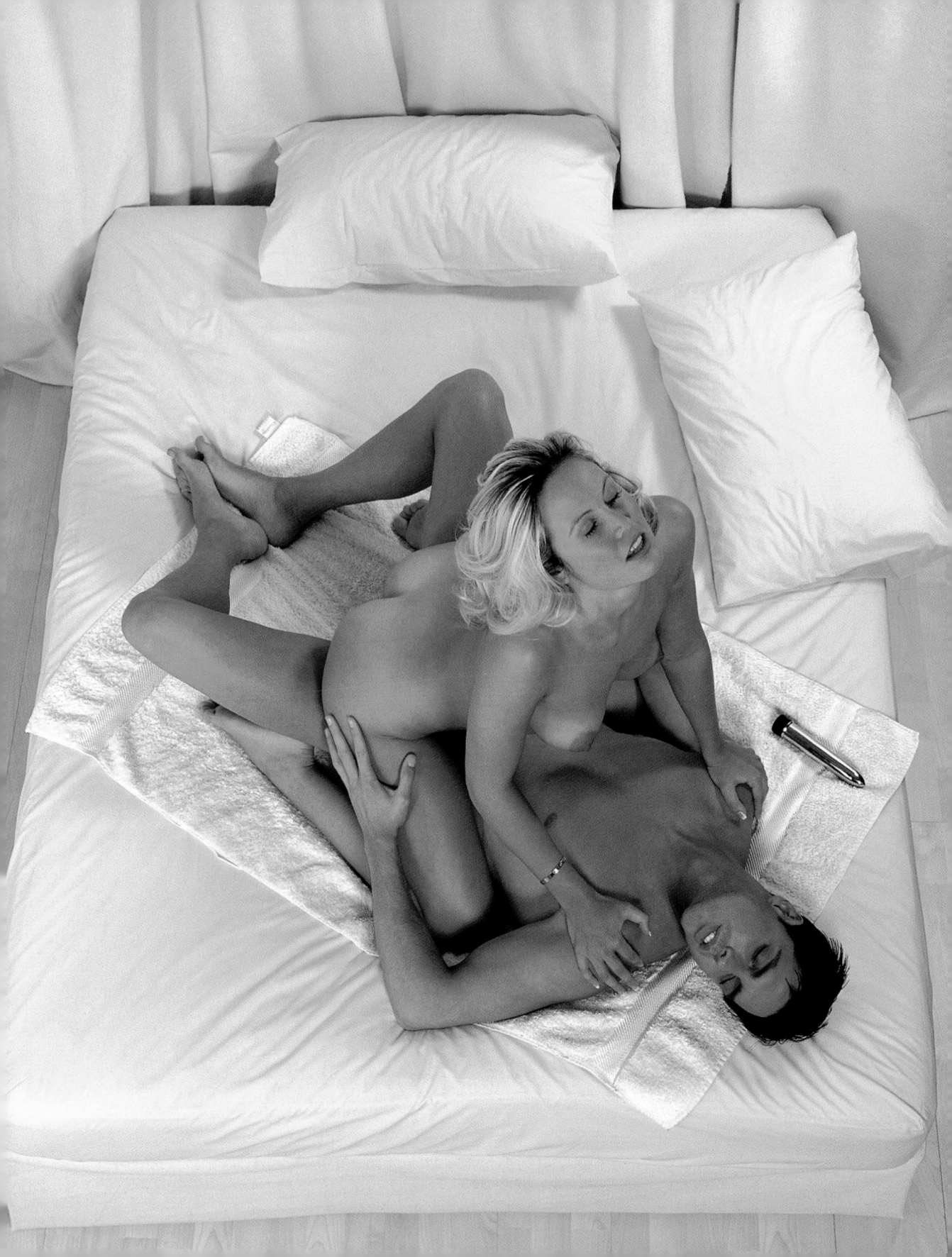

the blindfold: Next, help your partner to achieve this mental change of gear by whispering: 'Relax, let yourself go, forget the day, forget where you are, lose yourself, don't think about me, let your mind wander where it will and visit that secret erotic place only you know about and can enter', all the while making your caresses both more persistent and more teasing by slowing down your rhythm even further. Touch the side of the neck with tenderly applied feather-strokes from your finger-nails. Do the same to the sides of the breasts, inner thighs, buttocks and groins. Make the visits of your fingers to the genitals almost a rarity. Hint in the same subdued voice how it might be more fun for your partner to close his eyes, to see nothing, to float into darkness and focus on his dreams, and suggest he could find this easier if he borrowed your bedside blindfold.

caution: Since this is a 'a first time', be ready to switch the mood back to more conventional lovemaking if your partner requests it. Alternatively, you may now have them at your complete mercy and ready to enjoy a little more psychological pressure: 'Do you like me to touch you there?' you ask, as your fingers momentarily tantalise a nipple, or titillate a headstrong penile glans. 'Is it wonderful? Would you like more?'. 'Oh dear,' you say, 'it seems to be stopping. Look, it's stopped.' Follow this up with a cruel 'And would you be willing to pay to get it to start again?'

how to pay: This should also be suited to your partner's level of comfort with the overall game. Perhaps you will compel them merely to say 'I beg you to touch me there' or insist they use the word 'Please'. Payment can also be made by tolerating an ice cube pressed to the navel (or any other warm rosy section of anatomy) or receiving mild slaps on the buttocks, the number to be negotiated. Whatever is decided, remember to keep the price just a tad high – remember, the best caresses should always be stopped *before* the recipient expects them to vanish.

finally: When your partner has reached his 'point of no return', break off from the game and using hands, mouth, or genitals commence rapid and vigorous sex till he climaxes.

afterwards: Resume everyday roles, be loving and reassuring, be full of thanks and praise – and suggest you might be willing to be on the receiving end next time – if he dares …

CASE ONE

Mark, 28, Software dealer; Jane, 25, sales executive:

Mark and Jane have been living together for a little over three years and have a one-year-old child called Ellie. Jane experienced post-natal depression and found it difficult to resume interest in sex for months after the birth and while breast-feeding. The breakthrough came on the afternoon Mark ceased to be a complete gentleman and coaxed her into submitting to some pleasure which he warned her was unavoidable …

Mark is a really nice man – nice and chunky to look at, a bit like the movie actor Richard Dreyfuss – with prematurely grey hair and laughing eyes. He says: 'I was very sensitive to Jane being off sex. I'd read all the books explaining how hormonal changes happen after pregnancy and about the psychology of becoming a new family with extra responsibility. We used to spend ages in bed just lying there cuddling, or she'd finish me off by hand. But I wanted to see if she could respond too. So one evening, when we'd gone to bed early, I asked her to get under the covers, which I then tucked tightly in all round. Then I sat astride her chest with my head facing her feet trapping her arms by her sides. I leaned forward and began massaging her soles, nibbling and sucking her toes and getting her to lose herself in a rhythm of dreamy pleasure. Then I slowly worked my way up her body until I could find her clitoris. The position was a little awkward but I kept my legs firmly clamped on her hands and moved my tongue in time to some favourite soul records. She struggled – but I must have found an irresistible spot because suddenly she opened her legs wide and let me do anything I wanted … '

Jane is of medium height, dark, with a figure-of-eight, very feminine body. She has a pretty mouth that smiles easily now the depression has gone. 'I'm not sure I ever want another baby. I adore Ellie now and would gladly die for her if it came to it but at the time she seemed to ruin my sanity and destroy my sexual feelings. I did *not* want to know about intercourse. I've since wondered whether the desire would have returned anyway but when Mark dominated me that night and got me to be 'selfish' I really did start to come back to life. I'd been feeling really guilty about not fancying him. It was such a clever switch to make me *unable* to touch him back. I couldn't even see his face – so of course I drifted off into my dreams. My feet adore being stroked and if you've never had a pedicure – don't imagine you're qualified to comment! Purrfect!'

CASE TWO

Alexander, 36, Police officer; Mireille, 29, Lecturer:

Alex and Mireille have been seeing each other for seven months. French, competitive, middle class and very go-getting – neither has ever spent much time talking about sex. They got together, fell for each other then into bed enjoying the conventional routines. 'In France, we don't talk so much about these matters. We assume everyone is a wonderful lover simply by virtue of being French,' said Alexander. But, one evening after a succession of brandies in the forest cabin his family has owned for three generations, things began to change.

Alexander has a scar on his cheek that only makes his dark good looks slightly more mysterious. Tall and well-dressed he says the scar is *not* romantic – he fell off his roller skates as a child. But it was one of his first experiences of tolerating pain. The memory recurred when Mireille and he were making love: 'Mireille was giving me the most marvellous caresses on a kind of love seat for two people in the living room. I was very woozy from drink. I even think I snoozed for a couple of moments. When I woke up I found Mireille had secured my hands to some heating pipes high up on the wall. I was lying on my back with my arms spread in a sort of crucifix position.

Then she stood in front of me, killed the overhead lights so she was just backlit by a tablelamp. All I could see was the outline of this beautiful woman's body but not her face, no details. Then she walked towards me, slid her skirt up over her hips and offered me her sex. She came towards me, very provocatively, and stopped inches from my lips, kneeling across my body. But no matter how hard I strained or how much I hurt my wrists, I couldn't touch her. All I could do was smell that beautiful scent of a woman and I wept with frustration. And she wouldn't relent and refused to let me have her, even though I begged. She even laughed, then masturbated in front of me, then fell asleep herself! Never as a grown man have I been treated like that ... '

Mireille may appear bookish with her spectacles on but she is very warm, approachable and full of friendly charm. She has learned to be wary of men who make easy promises and has enjoyed running her own life since the divorce: 'I wanted to shock Alexander. He's such a powerful guy deciding who's free to come and go all day long. I suddenly had this hunch that he might enjoy knowing what it's like for all the criminals and illegal immigrants he deals with. I also loved showing him my body and telling him he *only* gets pleasure from it if I *allow* him to. I also loved taking my time because normally he turns me on so quickly I cannot savour the experience. It's not true, of course, that I was very cruel. He's forgetting quite how much he'd had to drink. He also fell asleep again. First thing in the morning I woke him up with oral sex and he was very satisfied. But I notice he now asks me if we can "play that game" again and I'm planning to become tougher.'

CASE THREE
Jenni, 31, Fashion designer; Raoul, 32, Lawyer:
Jenni and Raoul's happy marriage came under strain because Jenny was tiring of Raoul's very physical approach to sex. For Raoul, intercourse was like a passionate exercise, helping rid his body of everyday tensions. Sylvester Stallionesque. He didn't mind if the marriage carried on in the same routine forever. For Jenni, an artistic individual, sex was a means of reaching new moods and exploring her imagination. She had always enjoyed fantasising about her more aggressive side and was attracted to novel erotic ideas partly in response to recent trends in fashion. In bed, she began to want actual control. Raoul was initially confused by her new demands. He didn't understand what was wrong with the old ways since every time they had made love before Jenni had seemed to climax. Wasn't that the point of it all?

Jenni is just under 5' 10" with very white skin, high cheekbones and dramatic eyes. She wears her hair in a severe bob and looks masterful. 'I sometimes think Raoul has never recovered from discovering that women *can* have sex. He's bowled over by knowing that we have this potential ability to engage in sexual intercourse. It's as if he's still in awe of the vagina. He can't seem to understand that genitals are just genitals *unless* you think of a different way to handle them! I really don't mind if I never have straight intercourse again. But I would kill to be in bed enjoying intercourse with a man who could first tamper with my mind, either by submitting himself to me, placing himself under my control, or else having the magical power to take me over, and make me almost want to hurt myself with desire. Fortunately, Raoul is a learning person and I believe we're going to have a great deal more fun together … '

Raoul is the same height as Jenni but dark skinned with short wavy hair and long sideburns. He works out and keeps in shape by swimming every lunch hour: 'It took me a lot of grief and self-analysis before I came to realise Jenni meant what she said about our sex-life – that it would have to be different from now on, or at least for some of the time. All I heard when she first talked to me was criticism. I come from a culture where men are kings. We open doors for ladies, try to touch them on the bottom as they go past and then pretend nothing has happened. It was a big step to let Jenni tie me up and insult me to my face. But I have to say, although it made me angry at the time, I got completely focused and aroused and when finally *she* let me come, I practically hit the ceiling.'

CASE FOUR
Carrie, 29, Trainer; Steven, 33, Politician:
Carrie and Steven have been having an affair for five years. Carrie grew up in San Francisco where she ran rather wild from the age of 15 and had one unpleasant experience of being mugged by a man who sliced her halter top with a knife and fondled her breasts before taking her purse. This memory frequently feeds into her sexual fantasies. Later, she had a relationship with an older man of great wealth, who enjoyed using his money to control those around him. Steven comes from London, England. Before running across Carrie in California, he had never known a woman who could stand up to his sharp tongue and quick mind. For the first two years, their affair was conducted with more heat than light, always on the edge, with neither really sure of the other's commitment. Now they have 'become firm friends' who can still have a red-hot love life even after several years of intimacy. Their friends are jealous and would love to know the secret. It can now be told.

Carrie has a bird's nest of frizzy red hair, a round face, heavy curved eyebrows, big pouty lips and extremely long legs. If she wears high heels, all men feel small: 'I tend to divide my life into Before Steven and After Steven. He's what I've always wanted. He can accept the bits of my mind that have bothered all my other lovers. In the past, like a lot of women, I've been attacked physically. There was also a lot of stress with my Dad. As a result, my desires and memories aren't straightforward. I'm a curious mixture of the sweet and bitter. When I'm highly aroused, and

Steven is brilliant at tipping me over, I quickly disappear into a world where people are *not* just oh-so-nice and kind and reasonable. They're cruel too and it excites me to pieces. I call this mental place "sexland".'

Steven is tall and well-built with fine balding hair and a taste for power suits by G. Armani. He's well-known in his own country: 'I don't honestly know whether there's a speck of native sadism in me or whether Carrie provokes me into playing a game entirely for her benefit. Whatever the truth, I get this overwhelming urge to punish or restrain her, to make her take pleasure even if she doesn't want it, to force the pace, commence intercourse early (or delay it), to make her endure caresses that are rude or assaulting but which I ensure are very pleasant anyway, then to tease her till she begs me to make love again. The bottom line is always the same. I spend a lot of time stoking up her passion so that she has the most explosive orgasms possible. So who's really in charge? Me, the eager-beaver lover, or her, the woman who gets me to approach her body and soul in a totally different and fresh manner each time we meet? Last week, I kissed her for about 15 minutes in the kitchen until her face was red. Then I said I had to go to the bathroom and made sure she waited for another ten minutes before steaming her up again. She was furious but grateful in equal proportions.'

Of course, role play will seem meaningless if the acting is only skin deep. Without implying that women have a responsibility to educate men, the next chapter suggests ways in which you can ensure that your male companion is both involved and committed.

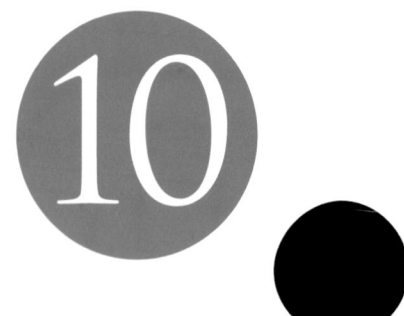

10.

TEACHING *intimacy* TO MEN

What's life without intimacy? It's probably a life without happiness and possibly a life where you often feel ill. Many of our clients feel that way. And it's very difficult to get them to see what intimacy is and isn't. Many have nice houses and cars, a nice life and nice clothes. Some are very wealthy. They have partners and people they call friends. They are slept with and they even have sex. But they don't get intimacy.

Some choose to be single. The single life may be what they want. Some are wary of commitment. Others put their chosen career or profession first. But they lack intimacy and they feel the effects of not having it. Others may be married. But the same applies. You can sit having dinner

HOW INTIMATE A LOVER ARE YOU?

❦ Can you talk about anything in bed?　　　　　　YES ☐ NO ☐

❦ Can you look into each other's eyes as you
love each other?　　　　　　　　　　　　　YES ☐ NO ☐

❦ Can you make love without intercourse?　　　　YES ☐ NO ☐

❦ Can you enter into each other's fantasies?　　　YES ☐ NO ☐

❦ Can you offer your lover sexual treats that
don't do anything for you?　　　　　　　　　YES ☐ NO ☐

If you score high on the YESs, you are a prize, an exceptionally intimate
lover. You are so comfortable with your sexuality that you can accept and
take part in any aspect of sex with your partner. You are a joy in bed
because you are responsive, imaginative, trusting and creative.

If you score more or less equally with the YES/NOs, join the club. You are
like most of us in that you can be highly intimate but possess sticking
points. You may long to act out fantasies but be scared that by doing so you
could lose either the fantasies or the partner. You may long to go completely
wild during sex but be just that bit too inhibited.

If you score high on the NOs you may need to shed inhibition, to give and
receive trust, to learn more about sex and to experiment with your partner
provided your partner feels safe. You are probably longing to be really
intimate with the person you adore but just don't quite know how – yet.

at some fancy restaurant enjoying the good life. Your partner can burble
charmingly about the events of the day. You can drive home in the latest
Jaguar with all the gadgets and open the door to your designer living
room snug with burglar alarms and deep welcoming sofas. But you still
feel lonely. You don't have any intimacy and you don't know how to get
it. And you don't know how to get it because you don't know what it is.

WHAT IS INTIMACY?

Writer Joel Levy offers this definition: 'Intimacy is a combination of
emotional warmth and openness, and a free and open flow of communication. It involves sharing, valuing your partner, knowing he values
you, and all the acts that make you feel close. But there is nothing
necessarily sexual about intimacy – it can also be the friendship and
trust you have with a platonic friend.'

In mental health terms, intimacy is about respecting another person's significance beyond their material and physical necessities. For example, you can't generate intimacy by lavishing hugely expensive gifts upon your partner. You will only succeed if the present is *also* personal and has sentimental value. Intimacy is about investing your private care, not your coins.

Nor is it just about sexual relationships and marriage. Intimacy can be about brief, everyday contact. You can spend all weekend with a lover and never feel he is even present in the room. He makes love to you by turning in a great performance but never opens himself up. 'I don't feel I know this man at all,' said one of our clients, 'Even though I can tell you how many moles he's got on his back.' But sometimes you can meet a friend in the street, stop for a quick coffee and feel completely re-energised and connected by the shared confidences, hurried efforts at joint problem-solving and the affection of mutual support. It took perhaps 13 minutes and nobody thought of removing a sock.

A similar level of intimacy can happen in therapy. You create an incredibly close relationship with a counsellor, who knows all your secrets and assists you through any and every crisis. But you may never even shake hands, let alone have a coffee together. The relationship is professional, non-physical but full of the sound of emotional barriers giving way. Even so, intimacy remains bigger than sex. After one client made a pass, the counsellor said; 'We are not going to have sex because I think it's more important to be here for you rather than take from you.' She said: 'You don't know what a relief it is to get all that out of the way.' Sometimes in circumstances such as these, intimacy prospers when sex is declined.

WHY IS INTIMACY SO IMPORTANT?

After food, intimacy is perhaps our biggest hunger. Intimacy matters because we are creatures who need approval, support and endorsement especially from those who seem similar to us. That's the way we grow up in families. That's the way our nervous system works. That's the legacy of 10,000 years of conditioning in small tribes and communities. Everything we do and have is social – even the words we use to speak were received from others. No man is an island – and no woman becomes Prime Minister without a little encouragement. If we really could 'do everything by ourselves' there wouldn't be any relationship problems in the world and far less mental illness. We would all become our own stimulating best friends.

If you don't believe me, try a simple experiment next time you go on holiday, or when you find yourself on a weekend course with people you like. By the last day I bet you will want to swap names and addresses with those you've met and plan some sort of future reunion. You are recognising that intimacy has been created and you are reluctant to let it go. We even tend to hold an alcohol-fuelled grief ceremony to cope on the final night.

The fact is that we all need to feel connected however much we deny or resist it. We like to think at least one close friend 'holds a file on us', to stay informed on our progress through life. It doesn't even have to be a friend. What are hairdressers and personal trainers for? These are a special class of folk who can actually take an interest, remember what page of the script we're on and see the world from our point of view. What men might dismiss as silly girlie chat is actually the lifeblood of intimacy. And they do exactly the same thing with barbers and taxi-drivers.

CAN YOU GENERATE INTIMACY IF IT'S MISSING?

Yes, look at Jenny and Michael. They've have been living together for 27 years with two children in college. Their partnership seems intimately happy though sex is not a priority. Jenny says lovemaking used to be frequent (every single day in Years 1 and 2). But after a couple of infidelities and a crazy time when nobody said anything their affair has evolved into something more like friendship – they are 'intimate friends'.

'We love each other. Mike is my best friend, my business partner, my mate. We are constantly affectionate, kiss and cuddle every day, touch, stroke and say tender words. What we have together is consideration, shared memories, great tolerance, forgiveness, the same sense of humour, two wonderful kids, a house with a garden we love and pleasure in each other's company...'

Mike says: 'I guess intimacy must include putting the other person first when the chips are down. You know, rushing to their side in a crisis. It means tolerating the times when Jenny is depressed and takes some of it out on me – and it means me knowing that that's what's happening, being able to recognise it and take the long-term view. It's like surviving the tantrums of your children – you don't like it – but you love them. And I love Jenny.'

'When we go away for weekends,' says Jenny, 'we do it for us, for the relationship. We also give each other presents. Nothing expensive – I'm a cheap date – just a book the other wants or sometimes even some information in a cutting from the newspaper. We remember things the other person has talked about. Or he'll take one look at my weary face and go out and do the supermarket shop on his own, then come home and cook. One of the reasons I feel like loving him is that he can read my moods.'

Behavioural psychologist Dr Robert Sharpe author of *How To Do A Good Deal Better With Others* suggests that intimacy requires a precise emotional skill: 'Can you look your partner in the eyes and say "I see you feel X about Y"?' If your husband walks in and says: 'Gosh you seem keen to have me home – is everything okay?' his behaviour at

THE INTIMACY FORMULA

- ❤ Remember your friend/lover's priorities
- ❤ Keep a rough idea of their schedule
- ❤ Ask about their moods and state of mind
- ❤ Predict to yourself what they are likely to be feeling
- ❤ Become a better, more active listener
- ❤ Show affection – small touches matter
- ❤ Be forgiving – learn to count to ten
- ❤ Be amusing – try to entertain and be funny
- ❤ Let someone have a go at you when they should
- ❤ Give appreciation – say thank you – take nothing for granted
- ❤ Keep saying what you like about them and why
- ❤ Disclose your own fears, worries and hopes
- ❤ Say sorry when you've screwed up

once will make you feel understood, accepted and encouraged. If he just grunts 'Hi', you will feel more isolated and if he ignores you – you'll feel diminished.

As we've already noted, Dr John Gottman in his recent research on what makes relationships work says that intimacy is actually constructed from all those little endearing acts that lovers spontaneously perform for each other when they first pair up but which over the intervening years get lost in the mid-life fog. Jenny making the effort to buy Mike the paperback he raved about at breakfast, he says, is one of the basic things which couples in successful partnerships do to foster intimacy.

CAN YOU TEACH INTIMACY TO MEN?

A famous, much married, actress once said: 'You know, it's women who are like dogs and men who are like cats. Not the other way round. Women are men's faithful friends. Men the ones who start rubbing your ankles when they want to get something. They're out roaming the town all night looking for a playmate. Women stay in guarding the house. Men are detached. If they find a better deal they take it. Women want the intimacy of familiar connections. The house catches fire, they'll be at home fighting the blaze or getting trapped inside.'

Okay, perhaps we shouldn't listen to the voice of prejudice with four ex-husbands as baggage. We've all known men who cling to their wives and women who act like sex kittens. But there's enough truth in the stereotype to put the question – why *do* women complain that men would sooner join the army than discuss their feelings.

Normal male behaviour does discourage the showing of emotion. Men have had centuries of locking antlers with their rivals so *don't* divulge secrets easily. In fact, normal male behaviour stretches off the graph until it's difficult to distinguish from mild forms of autism. Some men appear devoid of emotional needs. They get on with their lives whatever happens to them. Until it comes to ego.

This is where you could make the difference. As we've said, women probably require some level of intimacy in order to enjoy sex. Men require high self-esteem in order to risk intimacy. This often results in a deadlock, a cold war. But if you want to get your man to open his heart you *first* need to make him feel more important to himself. It's perfectly simple.

MEN ARE PRAISE-SEEKING MISSILES!

You don't even have to give them your body. Jenny, for example, doesn't. But the way to any man's heart generally lies through a subtle form of personal approval. It's not quite flirting, not really exaggerated flattery. Just an open appraisal: 'I like the look of you. I'd really want you if we could just settle a few of our differences and get them out into the open. Not only would I want you – I'd probably be all over you!'

And nor is this based on a lie because if you currently share your life with any man there's likely to be some sort of bond. What really turns a cold warrior into a friend is telling him the details of why he's lovable. Positive appreciation of his attractions – any attractions – is always more successful than negative criticism of his legendary failings. So if you want intimacy with your man, give him days and nights of encouragement.

CONCLUSION

And so back to the beginning. The purpose of this book is to offer insight from a man *and* a woman into the male sexual world. Men seem to invest a disproportionate amount of their personal identity in sexual success. Although possessed of the same number of emotions as women, they deploy them differently. Somehow, male love-life is connected to and separate from social emotions. Men need sexual friendship but are also highly threatened by it. They want to be close to individual women and yet fancy sex with women in the abstract. They are a bit of a puzzle to themselves as well as others.

Our one hope is that at the end of this volume you will now feel confident to offer and receive more sexual pleasure within a framework of mutual acceptance and understanding. Men don't wake up in the morning asking themselves 'How can I really make her life hell today?' They are trying to solve their problems as best they can. They are stuck with maleness as much as you are stuck in femaleness. The only way forward is through celebrating and negotiating the differences where they count – in bed, in dialogue, in love.

QUESTIONS TO ASK YOURSELF AT THE END

There are no correct answers to these questions. They have been devised to help you think more precisely about what you really expect from a loving sexual relationship:

1 If you had your time over again, would you pick the same partner?

2 Do you trust your partner concerning money? (Would you trust him to take the male contraceptive pill?)

3 If you had a penis for a day, would you study it, use it, share it or reject it?

4 If you thought your partner had another lover, would you confront her, confront him or ignore it?

5 Does your partner know your most erotic fantasy or is it secret?

6 Would you prefer a pleasant celibate millionaire or a lovable rogue with a golden cock and no cash?

7 Would you like to make love more or less often than you do?

8 What would make you dump your partner – obesity, baldness, impotence, bankruptcy, chronic illness?

9 Would you rather have an orgasm or a nice necklace?

10 Is your lover the man you wish to grow old with?

11 If your partner wanted to shave your pubic hair, would you let him? (Would you agree to be tattooed?)

12 If you found your partner applying lipstick, would you be amused or disgusted?

13 If you could change one aspect of your partner's lovemaking what would it be?

14 And how would you go about communicating that wish?

FURTHER READING

Bancroft, John. *Human Sexuality And Its Problems* (2nd Edition) (Churchill Livingstone, Edinburgh, 1989)

Brothers, Joyce. *What Every Woman Should Know About Men* (New York, 1981)

Carlson Jon. and Sperry, Len. (Eds) *The Intimate Couple* (Brunner/Mazel, Philadelphia 1999)

De Angelis, Barbara. *Secrets About Men Every Woman Should Know* (Thorsons, New York, 1990)

Deurzen-Smith, Emmy van. *Everyday Mysteries. Existential Dimensions Of Psychotherapy* (Routledge, London 1997)

Goleman, Daniel. *Emotional Intelligence* (Bloomsbury, London 1996)

Gottman, John. *Why Marriages Succeed Or Fail* (Bloomsbury, London 1997)

Hodson, Phillip. *Men: An Investigation Into The Emotional Male* (BBC, London 1984)

Hodson, Phillip. *What Kids Really Want to Know About Sex* (Robson, London 1993)

Hodson, Phillip. *The Cosmopolitan Guide To Love, Sex and Relationships* (Headline, London, 1997)

Hooper, Anne. *The Ultimate Sexual Touch* (Dorling Kindersley, London 1995)

Hooper, Anne. *The Thinking Woman's Guide To Love And Sex* (Robson Books, London 1983)

Hooper, Anne. *The Ultimate Sex Guide* (Dorling Kindersley, London 1992)

Kern, Roy, Hawes, E. Clair and Christensen, Oscar C. (Eds) *Couples Therapy: An Adlerian Perspective* (Educational Media Corporation, Minneapolis 1989)

Kramer, J and Dunaway, D. *When Men Don't Get Enough Sex And Women Don't Get Enough Love* (Pocket Books, New York 1990)

Janda, Louis H, and Klenke-Hamel, Karin E. *Human Sexuality* (D Van Nostrand Company, New York 1980)

Masters, William H. and Johnson, Virginia E. *Human Sexual Response* (Little Brown, Boston 1966)

Stubbs, Kenneth Ray. *Romantic Interludes: A Sensuous Lovers Guide* (Secret Garden, Larkspur 1986)

Wilson, Glenn and Nias, David. *Love's Mysteries: The Psychology Of Sexual Attraction* (Open Books, London 1976)

Wilson, Glenn. *The Secrets Of Sexual Fantasy* (Dent, London 1978)

Zilbergeld, Bernie. *Men And Sex – A Guide To Sexual Fulfilment* Souvenir Press, London 1978)

APPENDIX

If you'd like to email the author Phillip Hodson, or review any of his other work, please make contact via his website – **www.philliphodson.co.uk** Phillip is also Head of Media Relations for the British Association for Counselling (1 Regent Place, Rugby CV21 2PJ, 01788 550899 or contact **www.counselling.co.uk**), and Chairman-elect of the Impotence Association (PO Box 10296, London SW17 9WH, helpline 0208 767 7791 or contact **www.impotence.org.uk**). Phillip Hodson is also a Member of the British Association of Sexual and Marital Therapists (PO Box 62 Sheffield S10 3TL), and the London Marriage Guidance Council. (Anne Hooper can be reached at **www.annehooper.com**).

If you want to explore group or relationship workshops, or wish to develop your confidence or 'seduction' skills, please contact Phillip's colleague Peta Heskell who has wide experience and is retained by leading companies to help employees develop their team and inter-personal communication (Peta organises the 'UK Flirting Academy' on 0700 4354 784 or contact **www.flirtzone.com**)

If you'd like to find out more on the subject of male hormone replacement therapy, testosterone supplements or anti-ageing health strategy please contact Dr John Moran (Hormonal Healthcare, 30a Wimpole Street, London W1, 0207 935 4870) and/or Dr Michael Perring (Optimal Health of Harley Street, 114 Harley Street, London W1, 020 7935 5651 or contact **www.OptimalHealth.org.uk**

If you are interested in sexual politics, you may be interested in reaching the Sexual Freedom Coalition (PO Box 4ZB London W1A 4ZB, 0207 460 1979 or contact **www.sfc.org.uk**)